THE

OMEGA-3

PHENOMENON

The Nutrition Breakthrough of the '80s

THE

OMEGA-3

PHENOMENON

The Nutrition Breakthrough of the '80s

Donald O. Rudin, M.D., and Clara Felix

with Constance Schrader

RAWSON ASSOCIATES : New York

Library of Congress Cataloging-in-Publication Data

Rudin, Donald O.
The Omega-3 phenomenon.

Bibliography: p.
Includes index.
1. Omega-3 fatty acids—Therapeutic use.
2. Omega-3 fatty acids—Physiological effect.
3. Fish oils in human nutrition.   I. Felix, Clara.
II. Schrader, Constance.   III. Title.
RM666.045R83   1987   615′.34   86-42533
ISBN-0-89256-314-1

Published simultaneously in Canada by Collier Macmillan Canada, Inc.
Packaged by Rapid Transcript, a division of March Tenth, Inc.
Copy edited by Bob Oskam
Composition by Folio Graphics Company, Inc.
Designed by Jacques Chazaud

First Edition

Contents

PREFACE: The Inside Story—Never Again   *ix*

ACKNOWLEDGMENTS   *xvii*

PART I: Solving the Mystery of the Missing Nutrient—Eat Better to Feel Better   *1*

1. The Missing Nutrient   *3*
2. Nutritional History Repeats Itself   *6*
3. Omega Fats for Total Fitness   *8*
4. Fiber and Omega-3 Work Together   *26*
5. The Seven Factors That Affect Your Health   *30*
6. How Disease Develops   *33*
7. Health Benefits for the Omega-3 Program Volunteers   *43*
8. The Omega Complexion Connection   *50*
9. The Omega Topical Skin-Care Program   *58*
10. Omega-3 Nutrition for Men, Women, and Children   *61*
11. The Omega Factor in Breast-Feeding and Formula Feeding   *68*
12. Omega Case Histories: Mental Illnesses Respond   *76*
13. Omega Case Histories: Linseed Oil, Fish Oil, and the Heart   *82*

PART II: The Comprehensive Mega-Omega Supplement Program   *89*

14. The Omega Supplemental Program for Overt Illness   *91*

PART III: The Omega Diets: Getting It All Together *117*

15. The Omega EFA and
    the Three Traditional Food Groups   *119*

16. The Omega Shopping Guide   *130*

17. The Nutritionally Complete Everyday Omega Diet   *137*

18. Lose Weight and Keep It Off:
    The Three-Phase Omega Weight-Loss Program   *157*

19. The Gourmet-thin Omega Diet and Recipes   *184*

20. The Veggie-thin Omega Diet and Recipes   *208*

21. The Omega Antiallergy Diet   *225*

22. The Omega Mother-Infant Diet   *229*

23. Longevity and the Omega Antiaging Diet   *233*

24. Beware the Great American Experimental Diet   *238*

GLOSSARY   *241*

APPENDIXES

   A. Sources of Essential Fatty Acids   *247*

   B. For Those Who Want More Information   *257*

   C. The Modernization Disease Syndrome
      as Substrate Pellagra-Beriberi   *263*

INDEX   *277*

This book is dedicated to three pioneering reform nutritionists who have provided important evidence that the food we eat is the primary cause of the major illnesses in modern societies:

Dr. Abram Hoffer and his colleagues, who first proposed that mega-doses of B vitamins correct a widespread vitamin-resistant pellagra-form schizophrenia and other illnesses caused by modern dietary modifications.

Dr. T. L. Cleave and the British fiber theorists, who first established that a widespread dietary fiber deficiency in the modern diet contributes to a variety of bowel and bowel-related illnesses.

Dr. H. M. Sinclair, who first provided evidence that dietary Omega-3 essential fatty acid deficiency contributes to the development of cardiovascular disease.

And to Mr. David Shakarian, who pioneered mass marketing methods on behalf of dietary correction for the public health.

Preface
The Inside Story—
Never Again

The thesis of this book is simple: The evidence indicates that the bulk of illness in modern societies is the result of an unrecognized disease cluster that I call the "modernization disease syndrome." This cluster is caused by a multitude of food and dietary modifications interacting metabolically with stress and exercise deficiency. The food modifications have never been tested for their collective safety by health authorities, and it seems clear they interact in the body to produce a new kind of deadly *synergistic* malnutrition that is not caused by any one factor alone. The resulting biochemical disturbances center on a newly discovered fat-based regulatory system—the essential fatty acid–prostaglandin system—which regulates just about every body function. These disturbances, when playing against genetic variations, can then cause just about every illness known to medicine.

This modernization disease syndrome is the fatty cousin of the classical B-vitamin deficiency diseases of pellagra and beriberi, which once decimated entire societies with diverse illnesses in both East and West for more than 100 years, running into the early part of this century. These, too, were the result of food modifications, many of which continue to this day and to which we have added many others. Now we are succumbing to similar problems all over again and for the same reason. The ultimate cause is a persisting structural defect in our health care delivery system and health care regulation, which tolerates a medical monopoly over the whole of health care, even though our primary health problems are not medical but nutritional and life-style related. The result has been to put the health of our entire society at risk for the second time in the past 100 years.

As a researcher for thirty-five years—first in the Neurophysiology Laboratory of Anesthesiology at the Massachusetts General Hospital (within the Department of Pharmacology at Harvard Medical School) and later as Director of the Department of Molecular Biology in a clinical setting at the Eastern Pennsylvania Psychiatric Institute in Philadelphia—

I wondered if ignorance of the chemistry and nutrition of lipids (fats), one of the last great biochemical families to be worked out, might prevent us from recognizing a lipid deficiency/toxicity syndrome in man, even if we saw it. After all, deficiencies or excesses of every other major nutrient family—proteins, minerals, vitamins, and fiber—have been identified, after lengthy scientific investigations, as major public health hazards, despite considerable medical resistance to these findings. Could it be that the same great advances in technology that, in the hands of controlled biomedical science, have markedly reduced disease, might, in the hands of the food industry, cause equally marked but unrecognized nutritional disease? In particular, could they cause a lipid-centered malnutrition that could account for the modernization disease group and the fact that life expectancy in the mid-years has increased so little during the 100 years between 1850 and 1950, even though we have conquered the major killers of 100 years ago?

Such questions led me to evaluate the national dietary consumption figures and to compare them with disease incidences. The results show that modern food processing and food selection opportunities severely distort the availability of many essential nutrient and antinutrient families—especially limiting the Omega-3 essential fatty acids (EFA)—and that, wherever this occurs, the incidence of modernization diseases skyrockets. In fact, heart disease and certain cancers finally are being recognized as primarily linked to distortions of dietary fats. But what is most discouraging is that the heart and cancer experts rarely refer to one another's findings.

Why? Because this would make their two pet illnesses—heretofore considered unrelated—merely symptomatic variations of a single underlying nutritional disorder, the modernization disease syndrome. Most of our modern illnesses have been shown to increase ten- to a hundredfold about a decade after a society modernizes. My survey of contemporary national food consumption data shows that, compared to the typical unprocessed local diet consumed in 1850, today we consume, per capita, 100 percent more saturated fat and cholesterol, 250 percent more salt and refined sugar, and 1000 percent more "funny fats," the potentially dangerous isomers produced by hydrogenation. All of these act as "antinutrients," either blocking the use of our essential nutrients or increasing our requirement for them. But at the same time, we now consume 75 percent less dietary fiber, 50 percent less of certain minerals and B vitamins (especially B_6, and much less than that if one lives on soft drinks and fast foods), and 80 percent less of a critical essential fatty acid (EFA) family called Omega-3—the cold-climate ultrapolyunsaturates (including alpha linolenic acid, which I call the "nutritional missing link"). Moreover, the evidence discussed in this book indicates that the Omega-3 EFA are of such importance to primates and man that they could well be called the "primate essential nutrient." And yet, along with other essential nutrients, we have been systematically eliminating these for more than fifty years by food oil refining, cereal milling, and food selection patterns, none of which has ever been questioned by orthodox nutritionists and physicians.

Nutritionists and biochemists have overlooked this new illness syndrome because they think mainly in terms of single nutrient effects and single illnesses, now divided among a multitude of medical specialties. They have forgotten how clinically variable nutritional disorders such as beriberi and pellagra can be. Finally, the unique dependence of man on the Omega-3 EFA explains why the usual nutritional laboratory work on nonprimates has been irrelevant.

Nutritional synergism exists between most of the components of our diet. (That is, their combined effects are greater than the sum of their effects when considered individually.) For example, the EFA are protected from destruction in the body by the antioxidants consisting of vitamins pro-A, A, C, and E and selenium. In turn, the EFA are converted by the B vitamins into the fat-based regulatory system, including the prostaglandins, which regulate just about every body function at the tissue level. This nutritional synergism and the extensiveness of the regulatory systems affected by nutrition explain why, although no single food modification is alone responsible, a large number of small food modifications affecting different essential nutrients and antinutrients can interact to cause many different illnesses, depending on genetic susceptibility. It also explains why the therapeutic efficacy of all contemporary diets can be significantly enhanced by adding to them the nutritional missing link—the Omega-3 essential fatty acids. Because of this missing link, the full power of nutritional supplementation therapy—our primary line of treatment, or orthopharmacology—has not been realized until now, with the result that we too quickly turn to the therapeutic drugs of the physician—our secondary pharmacology.

Nutritional synergism also answers many of the major concerns of medicine and nutrition today. It explains why megadosing can be beneficial, at least for a while. It explains why so many different schools of nutrition claim similar benefits. For example, it explains why elevated serum cholesterol has been shown to be lowered by supplements of fiber alone, niacin alone, or Omega-3 EFA alone, and why all three taken together in combination with removal of saturated fat and other antinutrients will produce the greatest benefit. It explains why B vitamins and Omega-3 EFA supplements can separately correct various skin disorders. Similarly, it explains how, starting in the early 1950s, three different reform nutrition groups could correctly claim that dietary problems underlie our major illnesses.

T. L. Cleave and the British fiber theorists have provided strong evidence that a dietary fiber deficiency in modernized societies contributes to a variety of bowel and bowel-related illnesses, such as peptic ulcer, gallstones, irritable bowel syndrome (spastic colon or mucous colitis), diverticulitis, diabetes, and elevated serum fats.

H. M. Sinclair, J. Reed, and others, also of England, have provided evidence that an Omega-3 EFA deficiency is related to elevated serum cholesterol and cardiovascular diseases, including heart attacks, angina pectoris, and strokes, each of which is also a modernization disease.

Abram Hoffer of Vancouver has noted that our modern disease picture, ranging from schizophrenia to many physical illnesses, looks a great deal like old-fashioned B-vitamin-deficiency pellagra, except that it is vitamin-resistant—a "Hoffer pellagra." For this reason, Hoffer has been a major force behind the introduction of megavitamin therapy, at the same time urging a return to the consumption of nonprocessed, "live" natural foods, the goal being to achieve a diet approximating the traditional human diet, which, compared to our contemporary diet, contains vastly greater amounts of essential nutrients, including dietary fiber, Omega-3 EFA, selenium, and many B vitamins—as well as far less of the antinutrients, including saturated fat, "funny fats" (the isomers produced by hydrogenation), cholesterol, and sugar.

The fiber supplements recommended by Cleave, the Omega-3 EFA supplements recommended by Sinclair and Reed, and the niacin supplements recommended by Hoffer each reduce elevated serum fats (that is, fats in the bloodstream) when taken separately. I will show in this book that, especially when taken together and combined with a lowered intake of antinutrients, they also ameliorate many other modernization diseases as well. Clearly, supplementation programs must include both EFA families (Omega-6 and Omega-3), vitamin antioxidants (pro-A, C, E, selenium, cysteine, and minerals (macro and micro), as well as work toward a reduction of antinutrient toxicity effects produced by excessive consumption of saturated fat, cholesterol, sugar, salt, and "funny fats." In brief, we must return to the traditional natural diet if we are to prevent, ameliorate, and cure the modernization disease syndrome and its associated accelerated aging disease.

When it was discovered that modern steel roller milling of rice, wheat, corn, and other cereals contributed to beriberi and pellagra and that certain clinically recognized forms of these illnesses could be cured by specific B-vitamin supplements, experts assumed that they had learned all there was to know about the nutritional causes of these diseases. So they acquiesced in the continuation of the very milling practices that caused these illnesses in the first place, merely asking that millers add back vitamins B_1, B_2, and B_3, as though milling could not possibly destroy any other essential nutrients, unknown to the nutritionists of that time—or today, for that matter.

Now we learn that the germ removed by milling for the past 100 years or so also contains many other essential B vitamins, most of the essential minerals, and nearly all of the EFA. We have further discovered that milling also destroys dietary fiber, another essential dietary component. Moreover, as you will learn in this book, there are two families of essential polyunsaturates, not just one—the cold-climate Omega-3 EFA and the warm-climate Omega-6 EFA—and the former is systematically eliminated today by cereal refining/milling, oil refining/hydrogenation, and the consumption of warm-climate food oils, which lack the cold-climate Omega-3 EFA.

Elementary science requires that all food modifications from the traditional standard be outlawed, or at least contain warnings, until such time as they are proved safe and efficacious *in the context of our total diet over a period of at least several years, including the period of pregnancy.*

As a consequence of the unscientific approach tolerated by the medically dominated FDA and orthodox nutritionists, who have a real conflict of interest with respect to nutritional treatment, we not only continue to refine our cereals mechanically but have gone on to refine our cooking oils chemically through hydrogenation, thereby contributing to the destruction of 80 percent of the cold-climate Omega-3 EFA. We have also introduced isomers (funny fats) through hydrogenation at ten times traditional intake levels (which block the use of 20 to 40 percent of certain fatty acids). FDA regulations have made health-giving fish oils economically unprofitable for fish packers to use. And we have destroyed 80 percent of essential dietary fiber. To all this must be added the synergistic effects of our vastly increased consumption of both fatty beef and Omega-3–deficient southern foods (corn, peanuts, warm-climate wheat, cashews, sesame seeds) and food oils (corn, safflower, peanut, coconut, and a number of others). Meanwhile, we overlook the Omega-3–rich cold-climate oils and foods, including northern cereal grains, flaxseed, soy, walnuts, wheat germ, chestnuts, and northern beans, as well as fish and their oils.

Orthodox nutritionists go on glibly calculating how eating fast foods will increase this essential nutrient and reduce that one, when in fact they do not even know if they have a complete list of essential nutrients and antinutrients. Consequently, they never know how many essential nutrients they have failed to evaluate. Above all, they have never gotten around to demanding the simplest test of what they have wrought— namely, how well a colony of primates (our closest biological relatives) would fare on the ordinary supermarket diet on which nearly all of us live all our lives. From the evidence presented in this book, I freely predict that if a colony of monkeys were placed on the same supermarket diet we live on today, that colony would, within a few years, come down with all the modernization diseases, while a control group living on nonprocessed indigenous foods would not.

In my opinion, the current universal medical teaching asserting that workers in the United States, Holland, and Japan (Goldberger, Eijkmann, and Takaki) solved the problem of beriberi and pellagra around the turn of the century is wrong. What they solved was the B-vitamin deficiency form of these problems while leaving unidentified the much broader fat-centered deficiency-toxicity form that accounts for the bulk of disease today in modernized societies. In my opinion, *the medical profession has been misdiagnosing and mistreating the bulk of its cases for fifty to a hundred years or more.*

The Omega-3 essential fatty acids—the cold-climate ultrapolyunsaturates that come mainly from northern plants and fish—turn out to be the essential nutrient especially required by humans. They are also the unique factor in the cod liver oil supplements of our youth. Consequently, the facts recounted in this book can be viewed as reintroducing and scientifically updating the old-fashioned cod liver oil regimen. This is accomplished by using high Omega-3 foods and purified supplements, including linseed oil, which are appropriate for temperate and cold climates, in particular using these as therapeutic supplements for short periods of time in conjunction with antioxidants and other cofactors in the treatment of overt illness.

In support of this line of reasoning, I have conducted a new kind of clinical pilot study in forty-four patient volunteers over a period of several years. This study followed each case intensively over two to three years and, at the same time, cut across virtually the entire spectrum of medical specialties, both physical and mental. Consequently, what I am presenting here is not the usual statistical study of large numbers of patients all belonging to a single symptomatic disease group and studied by one specialty or another, but *an entirely new kind of individually intensive cross-specialty diagnostic and therapeutic investigation.*

The study used supplements of food-grade linseed oil, a high Omega-3 oil from plant sources. It was routinely used as a cooking oil and medicinal remedy in northern Europe until it was displaced by low Omega-3 EFA southern and hydrogenated oils following World War II. Linseed oil can be viewed as an approximate alternative to cod liver oil (very high in vitamin A) and other fish oils. However, only plant oils such as linseed oil contain alpha linolenic acid (ALA), which alone manipulates certain body enzymes. The fish oils lack this essential fatty acid but uniquely contain higher Omega-3 EFA, which manipulate other related enzymes. As a result, the plant and fish Omega-3 EFA can have different therapeutic effects, as I discuss later in this book.

So that spontaneous remission and placebo effects could be excluded, I accepted cases for study only if the individuals had long-term chronic illness that had failed to respond adequately to extensive orthodox medical treatment. In addition, the patients were mostly professionals who did not fit the placebo reactor personality profile. I also often cycled the patients off and on the linseed oil supplement or substituted low Omega-3 oils (safflower or corn) and found that improvement varied accordingly. Double blinds were impractical in this pilot study, especially since taste differences in the oils are marked. Finally, once improvement was seen with the oils, the other dietary corrections and vitamin supplements noted above were introduced if the patients were not already on them as part of their previous treatment, which was left untouched.

The clinical results can only be called spectacular. In addition to ameliorating many specific modern illnesses, both physical and mental, the findings also indicate that the stamina, vigor, and feelings of mental equanimity and well-being can be restored to many people who have been underperforming for many years, often without fully realizing it. Other reform nutritionists who have informally evaluated the regimen in their own practices for one to two years tell me they are seeing similar major benefits. Of course, formal confirmatory trials are needed. Nevertheless, the implications are clear, and I would consider it imprudent not to make the findings public at this point.

Fish oil supplements act like linseed oil. (Each has certain advantages and disadvantages, which I will discuss later in the book.) Some subjects report further improvement as the result of adding evening primrose oil, a relatively highly unsaturated form of Omega-6 EFA. The goal is to correct the basic diet and, when needed, to fine-tune the ratio of the oils used as supplements to fit each person's specific nutritional needs. Just as a single nutritional distortion can induce many different illnesses in different people because of differences in genetic susceptibility, so people can have varying requirements for different nutritional supplements, especially if they are ill. In that event they have reduced regulatory capacity. In some cases, improvement can be seen within hours or, more often, weeks. Other benefits take four to six months. Of course, severe cases may have suffered irreversible damage, in which case they cannot respond at all.

Because the modern diet has never been adequately tested as a whole for its safety against the only standard we have—the traditional local unprocessed diet—we can realistically call the average everyday diet "The Great American Experimental Diet." It requires that we all eat defensively in what amounts to a nutritional "Wild West," at least until such time as we develop adequate national food and health care policies. But as individuals we cannot wait either for long-term social reforms or for the results of long-term scientific tests. We must act prudently here and now, to take care of ourselves on the basis of considerable available evidence. Hence, the writing of this book, which brings together for the first time in one place the total nutritional story of our day.

These are important matters. The evidence indicates that our modern life-style diseases are our primary public health hazard, costing us more than any world war and now putting our society at risk in many unrecognized ways, extraclinical and social as well as clinical. Conversely, intelligent action can bring rewards exceeding those resulting from Pasteur's discovery of the cause of infectious disease and from Goldberger's discovery of the cause of classical pellagra as a B-vitamin deficiency disease.

I think that modern nutritional deficiencies may account for over half of all disease. But I also think there are—and have seen—wonderful cures and vigorous good health when adequate nutrition, through supplements and diet, is part of a healthy life-style. That is why I've written this book.

Part I discusses modern food technology—growing, packaging, and distribution—which has been a very mixed blessing, if a blessing at all. Several chapters deal with the growing realization of the potential problems associated with a manipulated food supply. Part I also shows how the newly discovered "nutritional missing link" (Omega-3 polyunsaturated fats) interacts in the body, providing promise of a healthier and longer life.

Part II provides the Mega-Omega Supplement Program, the first comprehensive supplement program for ameliorating overt illness.

Part III supplies the first truly comprehensive diets—Omega diets—designed for everyday living, obesity, allergies, fertility, pregnancy, infancy, and old age.

Donald O. Rudin, M.D.
Bryn Mawr, Pennsylvania
Spring 1987

Acknowledgments

The work on which this book is based was initiated at the Eastern Pennsylvania Psychiatric Institute. Shortsighted governmental support policies led to its disruption as it was about to reach fruition. The work was saved by grants from the Huxley Institute for Biosocial Research, Boca Raton, Florida, Dr. Abram Hoffer, founder and honorary President emeritus, and Mr. Ben Webster of Toronto, Canada, former Chairman of the Board of Trustees; by National Grocer's of Canada, Mr. John Shipton, President; and by General Nutrition Corporation of Pittsburgh, Pennsylvania, Mr. Bart Shakarian, formerly Vice-Chairman of the Board, and Dr. David Walsh, President of Manufacturing, then Vice-President of Research and Development. To these critically important backers, I express my deep appreciation for their support of the work.

My colleague and collaborator, Joan Rudin, has carried the burden of developing and testing the numerous menus and recipes, compiled the tables of food and food oil sources of EFA in Appendix A, and has contributed in many other ways, as have my colleagues Dr. Curt Dohan and Dr. Regina Flesch.

I am especially indebted to my coauthor, Ms. Clara Felix, and my collaborator, Ms. Constance Schrader, for making this complicated matter intelligible. Our editor, Ms. Grace G. Shaw, made many important editorial contributions. We thank our publishers, Ms. Eleanor S. Rawson and Mr. Kennett L. Rawson of Rawson Associates, for their steady encouragement, and my agent, Mr. Dominick Abel, for bringing us all together.

Part I

Solving The Mystery of the Missing Nutrient— Eat Better To Feel Better

1

The Missing Nutrient

edical research is a lot like detective work. The researcher seeks to resolve a health mystery, patiently follows leads . . . sometimes for years. However, the key to the puzzle can still elude you. In a novel, the mystery is solved at the end, the baffling threads woven neatly together. In medical research it seldom happens that way; the biggest problem may be to prove that a crime has been committed. And that is exactly the case with modern diseases.

Nobody seemed to notice that a crime had been committed: It was the case of the missing nutrient. The nutrient was essential; it was a nutrient we human beings needed in order to stay healthy. It started to disappear from our diet about seventy-five years ago and now it is almost gone. Only about 20 percent of the amount needed for human health and well-being remains. The nutrient is a fatty acid so important and so little understood that I call it "the nutritional missing link."

Can diet affect your total health?

The big killers in our country once were infectious diseases. Pneumonia, tuberculosis, diphtheria, typhoid fever, and smallpox were some of the worst. With the recent advances in medicine, sanitation, and public health we have won freedom from most of these deadly infectious epidemics. But we were cheated—a series of new plagues hit us. I call them "modern maladies" because they've increased with the sale and distribution of certain foods—along with the growth of food technology—since before the beginning of this century. Diabetes, cancer, heart disease, stroke, and obesity are at the top of the list, but also included are arthritis, allergies, irritable bowel syndrome, celiac disease, cystic fibrosis, anxiety-depression, hyperactivity, and schizophrenia.

What accounts for such a sharp rise in these disorders? I think the answer lies, to a large extent, in the significant changes in our diet that took place at the same time these diseases manifested themselves, starting when American diets changed from a rural-local food-supply focus to a

3

national food-supply chain of highly processed and imported foods. As food processing techniques depleted our food supply of vitamins, fiber, and other essential nutrients, food maladies became rampant.

Modern food processing problems are recognized by experts

Reform nutritionists and physicians who recognized these changes for the worse include Adelle Davis, T. L. Cleave, Denis Burkitt, Abram Hoffer, H. M. Sinclair, and many others. Their research and writing sparked a phenomenal grass roots movement. Millions of people are now aware of the logical connection between the foods they eat and the health problems they suffer.

Our modern food-related diseases, however, are still out there. As a researcher with thirty-five years experience, I followed a hunch: that something was missing from the average American diet—a special group of fats called Omega-3 fatty acids. It was one of the two families of fats absolutely essential to human life, and my survey showed the dietary availability of Omega-3 declining to only 20 percent of the level it held in traditional diets a hundred years ago.

Omega-3: The missing nutrient

Food-grade linseed oil and fish oils are the best sources of this special fat—Omega-3 essential fatty acid—which modern food destroys. But its depletion went unrecognized. Although in the current period of nutrition consciousness, everyone is enthusiastic about restoring nutrients to the diet, until recently Omega-3 was being ignored.

One method of scientific investigation is to speculate "What if?" What if the Omega-3 fats were restored? I worked in a clinical setting, and I knew that most studies cost millions of dollars and take years to get funded and launched, so many valuable studies just never happen. So, I reasoned, why not set up a small but representative pilot experiment, using volunteers/patients suffering from chronic ailments that are not being cured by current conventional treatment. Then add the missing Omega-3 oils to their diet and see what happens.

The forty-four-patient study

The study I set up included forty-four persons. I set several basic criteria for the patients to be included in the study. I looked for:

- People who had had one or more chronic complaints for a year or more
- Those who had not gotten well with the available traditional medical treatment or even with traditional nutritional therapy

- People who were not placebo reactors, e.g. tough-minded professionals. The kind of patient who is going to feel better after several days on any medication was not the right type for this study.
- Patients with a wide variety of common illnesses

Several years have passed since my forty-four-person experiment began. I've witnessed dramatic changes in the forty-four people who participated in this first pilot study of the missing fatty acid. What was most exciting was the amelioration of the symptoms of many seemingly different diseases, as well as a lifting of chronic fatigue and the increased sense of well-being that have become a hallmark of the treatment. My hunch about a missing nutrient—Omega-3—had been proven correct. It was a simple experimental study, and it worked. (If you are interested in the controls I used, see the Preface.)

I had done for my patients what any good mechanic should do for a car: I changed their oil.

Primate Needs for Fatty Acids Are Proven in Laboratory Test

Here is the story of an important but overlooked nutrition experiment using monkeys, primates with diet needs similar to man's:

Eight young capuchin monkeys placed on a laboratory diet with corn oil providing the only fat available all became sick within two years, although the diet in this 1970 British experiment was supposed to provide every nutrient requirement. Corn oil, with plenty of the Omega-6 essential fat linoleic acid, is routinely given in standard diets for laboratory rats and mice and was used in this study. The signs of fatty acid deficiency do not develop in subprimates—the rats and mice—on this diet.

But the monkeys developed dermatitis, diarrhea, and dementia on a diet on which mice thrive. Two capuchins suffered long bouts of diarrhea from an intestinal inflammation, and two other animals became psychotic, gnawing savagely at their own bodies, creating open, infected sores. All the monkeys developed dandruff and patchy hair loss. Clearly something was very wrong.

The surviving monkeys all recovered only two months after being provided nutrient supplements of linseed oil. The tiny amount of Omega-3 in corn oil might have been enough for rats and mice, but it clearly was not enough for the monkeys—and it is not enough for human beings either. When human societies go on similar modern diets, which today's nutritionists claim to be healthful, they get the same diverse array of illnesses those monkeys did. When modernized societies go "native" (during wartime), their modern illnesses disappear, just like those in my patient study group.

2
Nutritional History Repeats Itself

I set up my pilot forty-four-patient study because I wanted to test my theory that a new kind of epidemic of modern malnutrition was affecting America. Here are the stories of two other mysteries that parallel the mystery of the missing Omega-3 nutrient afflicting Americans today.

Beriberi

More than a hundred years ago, machine-polished white rice replaced unprocessed brown rice as a staple food throughout the Orient—Japan, India, Sumatra, and most of Indochina. The reason for change was simple: White rice kept better. White rice can be stored for months or years with little signs of deterioration.

Using steel rollers, the machine-milling process scraped off the outer husk of the rice to create a clean, white grain of rice. The discarded outer husk of rice material contained most of the grain's vitamins and minerals. Without this source of nutrients, native diets became deficient in thiamine (vitamin B_1). The deficiency led to an epidemic of beriberi that killed or crippled people for almost 200 years.

In "dry" beriberi, nerves degenerate and muscles waste. Paralysis starts in the legs and spreads over the whole body, and there may be severe psychosis. In "wet" beriberi, victims swell with trapped fluids and eventually suffer congestive heart failure. The symptoms mimic many diseases. The proof that they were symptoms of one disease, beriberi, and caused by a missing nutrient began to be apparent about the turn of this century, and the suspicion was definitely confirmed in the late 1930s. Thiamine (vitamin B_1) was synthesized in laboratories, and when it was introduced into the diet, many crazed and disease-weakened patients enjoyed miraculous recoveries.

A mystery solved.

Pellagra

The name *pellagra* is derived from two Italian words meaning "rough skin." Pellagra affects more than the skin; it runs a gamut of mental and physical illness. Diarrhea, dermatitis, and dementia (the "three D's") are some of the symptoms, just as they were symptoms in the laboratory experiment with the capuchin monkeys.

The mouth and tongue become bright red and ulcerated. Sometimes the sores extend into the digestive tract, producing swelling, pain, diarrhea, and constipation. The skin may develop a scaly dryness or redden, looking wind-chapped, or become permanently scarred and thickened. Fatigue, headache, weakness, arthritis, and tinnitus (a whistling or ringing sound in the ears) are also common physical symptoms.

The mental symptoms can range from irritability, nervousness, and depression to severe neurosis and psychosis. Pellagra victims filled insane asylums in our country early in this century, and in the first decade the disease was epidemic. It particularly affected poor families of sharecroppers and millhands. Hardest hit were women of childbearing age and children between the ages of two and ten.

Most of the people afflicted existed on a limited and deprived diet of refined corn meal, corn grits, corn syrup, a little lard, corn or cottonseed oil, and biscuits made from white flour. The victims seldom could afford milk, eggs, meat, or fish.

Although it was not known in North America at the time, the natives of Mexico and Central America who had subsisted for generations on a diet based on corn, had traditionally treated the corn with lime. Niacin—an important B vitamin—is present in corn, but in a form that is unavailable unless the corn is first treated with an alkali such as lime. Once niacin was isolated and put back in the diet, many pellagra sufferers recovered, but by no means all.

Another mystery solved.

3

Omega Fats for Total Fitness

Fat has a bad reputation it doesn't fully deserve. To many people the only association is with being overweight or obese. However, you cannot ignore the fact that your body needs certain fats for good health, and fat is also satisfying and filling. *You should eat some fat*—what matters is how much and what kind of fat you eat.

Don't be afraid of fat

Most nutrition and health experts agree that Americans eat too much total fat. We have one of the highest fat diets in the world. In a recent report the Food and Nutrition Board of the National Academy of Sciences noted that during this century the average fat intake has risen from 32 to about 42 percent of total calories consumed. This increase is attributed mainly to the use of fats and oils in cooking and to the increase in meat consumption. As a guideline, it was suggested that total fat intake not exceed 30 percent of total calories a day, particularly in diets below 2,000 calories. The board especially recommended lower consumption of saturated fatty acids such as those from animal products, limiting them to 10 percent of total calories.

Many nutritionists, myself included, would like to see the following proportion of foods in the average diet:

- 15 percent of calories from protein products
- 30 percent from fats
- 55 percent from carbohydrates (particularly complex carbohydrates)

Even people on weight-loss diets should get at least 25 percent of their calories from fats. Fats will lessen craving for food, because they move slowly through the digestive system, which keeps hunger pangs from recurring too soon. Meals low in fat can leave you feeling hungry very soon after leaving the table.

Body uses for fat

Fats—like carbohydrates, proteins, and alcohol—are sources of energy or calories. The body needs fuel to function, and fats are the most concentrated source of food energy. They provide 9 calories for every gram of food, compared to only 4 calories per gram from either protein or carbohydrates.

The body uses whatever fat it needs for energy (or calories), but excess fat does not simply disappear. It is stored in various parts of the body. Some fat is found in blood plasma and other body cells; the largest amount, by far, is stored in the body's adipose (fat) cells. These fat deposits not only store energy but also help to insulate the body and to support and protect body organs. Fats also serve as carriers for the fat-soluble vitamins—A, D, E, and K—and aid in their absorption from the intestine.

All fats are not the same

All fats are composed of the same three elements as carbohydrates: carbon, hydrogen, oxygen. However, fats have more carbon and hydrogen and less oxygen in their molecules than do carbohydrates. This gives them a higher fuel value. It is this difference that explains why fats supply more than twice as many calories as carbohydrates.

Fats in foods are mixtures of saturated and unsaturated fatty acids. In general:

- Saturated fats are solid at room temperature, e.g., beef and lamb fats, suet, and some dairy products.
- Unsaturated fats are liquid at room temperature and are called oils. Included among these are corn, cottonseed, soy, linseed, wheat germ, and walnut oils. (Coconut and palm kernel oils are saturated fats—they are solid at room temperature.)

Shortening and margarine are saturated fat products that have had hydrogen added by a process called hydrogenation. It saturates the oil and gives it a longer shelf life.

Omega-3 and Omega-6 EFA

Fats in food supply essential fatty acids, which are of major importance to human nutrition. They are:

- Essential to children for proper growth
- Needed to prevent drying and flaking skin
- Used to perform various metabolic roles
- Indispensable in the structure and functioning of cell membranes

Fats Under a Microscope

Most fats are compounds of fatty acids. Fatty acids are straight chains of carbon atoms ranging in number from two to twenty or more. Those above ten are called "long chain fatty acids." Each of these carbon atoms is linked to hydrogen atoms. The number of carbon and hydrogen atoms in a fatty acid, along with the different combinations of fatty acids found in a particular fat, determine how the fat will look and taste.

Saturated and Unsaturated

Fatty acids are either *saturated* or *unsaturated*. These terms refer to the number of hydrogen atoms attached to the carbon atoms in the fat molecule. When all the carbon atoms within the chain are linked to hydrogen atoms at all possible positions, the fatty acid is considered "saturated"—filled with hydrogen. When they are not, the fatty acid is "unsaturated"—there is a double bond between adjoining carbons instead.

Polyunsaturated fats have more than one instance of a double bond between carbon atoms. Linoleic acid, which has two double bonds, is the most common polyunsaturated fatty acid in food.

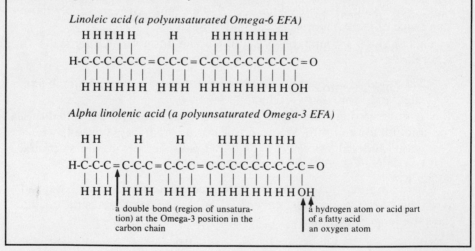

Linoleic acid (a polyunsaturated Omega-6 EFA)

Alpha linolenic acid (a polyunsaturated Omega-3 EFA)

a double bond (region of unsaturation) at the Omega-3 position in the carbon chain

a hydrogen atom or acid part of a fatty acid
an oxygen atom

• Regulators of cholesterol metabolism
• Raw material for hormone-like substances regulating nearly all body processes

The fats described as "essential fatty acids" are called that because they are necessary in the diet—they *must be* obtained from foods, since the body cannot produce them independently and yet cannot do without them. The amount of essential fatty acids (EFA) needed is small. But even though it is small, the average person still doesn't get an adequate amount.

Because corn and other vegetable oils used in the United States are particularly rich in linoleic acid, it is easy to get enough of this essential fatty acid in your regular diet. For example, a tablespoon of corn oil provides more linoleic acid than is needed by most people in a day. However, there is another type of EFA, the Omega-3 EFA, and we don't get a sufficient amount of this type essential fatty acid in our diets.

What is Omega-3 EFA?

Omega-3 refers to a group of fatty acids found in seafood and many cold-climate plants. Most vegetable oils we use today have a high content of the group of polyunsaturated fats called Omega-6 fatty acids. But most vegetable oils in use today have very little Omega-3 polyunsaturated fat, even though both groups are essential for good nutrition.

The work that is done by essential fatty acids (EFA) in our bodies— from assuring growth in children to maintaining cell membranes and producing special hormone-like substances (prostaglandins)—cannot be done by Omega-6 alone; Omega-3 EFA are also needed. It now appears that for many purposes Omega-3 EFA actually do a much better job than Omega-6. The best job is done when they are combined in the right proportions. Finding the best balance between Omega-3 and Omega-6 EFA can make a big difference in your total health.

Why Omega-3 and Omega-6?

The difference between the Omega-3 and Omega-6 EFA is that the EFA belonging to the Omega-3 family are more polyunsaturated than those belonging to the Omega-6 family. (*Omega,* the last letter in the Greek alphabet, refers to the last carbon in the chain (at left in the diagram on page 10).

An Omega-3 essential fatty acid is one in which the unsaturation (indicated by a double bond between two carbons) begins only three carbons in from the Omega carbon, while an Omega-6 EFA is one in which the unsaturation begins six carbons in from the end. As a result, the Omega-3 EFA have more regions of unsaturation along the chain than do the Omega-6 EFA. In fact, the lowest member of the Omega-3 family, called alpha linolenic acid, has three regions of unsaturation or double bonds. Other Omega-3 members have four, five (EPA, or eicosapentaenoic acid), and six (DHA, or docosahexaenoic acid). In contrast, the lowest member of the Omega-6 family, called linoleic acid, has only two regions of unsaturation, while the other members have three (GLA, or gamma linolenic acid) and four (AA, or arachidonic acid).

Why fats from cold climates are different

These differences are important chemically and physiologically, as additional double bonds make an EFA much more liquid at a given temperature. Northern plants produce more Omega-3 compared to the Omega-6 EFA in response to cold weather, since Omega-3 EFA keep cell membranes fluid, permitting them to function instead of freezing and fracturing. In contrast, southern plants produce very little Omega-3 but a great deal of Omega-6 EFA.

For this reason, I call the Omega-3 EFA the "*ultra*polyunsaturates" and refer to the better-known Omega-6 EFA as the "*regular* polyunsaturates."

What foods are rich in this vital Omega-3?

It all begins with plants and, in the ocean, plankton, a microscopic class of ocean plants that are at the base of the marine food chain. Plankton manufacture large quantities of the polyunsaturated essential fatty acid alpha linolenic Omega-3. Your body cannot manufacture this type of fatty acid, although you need it.

Fish—big fish and little fish, freshwater fish and saltwater fish—feed on the vegetable plankton and in that way get a rich supply of alpha linolenic Omega-3 fatty acids. From this they then build up two additional types of Omega-3 fatty acids found in seafood: docosahexaenoic acid (DHA) and eicosapentaenoic acid (EPA).

These are needed in the human body, and they work faster and better than regular Omega-6 vegetable oils to keep blood thin, to make body functions work better, and to prevent blood clots that would develop because of sticky blood platelets.

Linseed oil and Omega-3

Fish oils do not supply the simpler alpha linolenic acid, which has special functions. Nutritional linseed oil, made from flaxseed and available at most health foods stores, is very high in Omega-3 EFA and especially alpha linolenic acid. Although linseed oil has been used for centuries as a food and cooking oil, it is not as popular in America as some other vegetable oils. However, this oil is amazing in many ways. It is 60 percent Omega-3. This makes it an ideal oil for cooking and for supplementing your diet, to be sure that you get all the Omega-3 you need. Walnut, soybean, and wheat germ oil also are high in Omega-3 and can be used for food and cooking or as supplements, but as linseed oil is the highest in Omega-3, it is the best *plant* oil for therapeutic supplementation.

Linseed oil from plants, fish oils, and cod liver oil all supply large amounts of Omega-3 EFA. However, they supply different members of the Omega-3 family, and linseed oil has the following advantages in preventing and ameliorating illness:

1. Unlike fish oils, which are high in EPA and DHA, linseed oil is the only source of large amounts of alpha linolenic acid, ALA. This is the basic Omega-3 EFA—the body cannot make it—and the *only* one affecting certain enzymes regulating the production of specific types of prostaglandins. From ALA the body can then normally make the EPA and DHA found in fish oils. Fish oils also contain relatively high concentrations of vitamin A, which is toxic in large amounts. We limit cod liver oil intake to one teaspoon per day because of its high vitamin A content.

2. Linseed oil and the flaxseed from which it is made have been used for cooking and as a health remedy since the days of classical Greece and Rome. Until World War II, freshly squeezed linseed oil was delivered weekly to homes in northern Europe as a cooking oil, especially during Lent. Flaxseed is one of the unique ingredients of Roman bread, which is now coming on the market as a result of the work reported in this book (e.g., from Natural Ovens of Manitowoc, Wisconsin). Some families have a tradition of spreading a teaspoon of flaxseed over their breakfast cereal.

3. Linseed oil is far more palatable than fish oils, especially when taken in large therapeutic quantities and, unlike fish oils, it can be used for cooking and in salad dressing (see recipes), which provide easy ways to take large doses when needed.

4. Linseed oil is less expensive—it costs just a few pennies a day—than fish oil capsules (which cost 25¢ or more per day in comparable doses). Like fish oils, linseed oil can lower serum cholesterol and correct many other problems.

5. Only linseed oil has been extensively tried in clinical pilot studies (by myself and other reform nutritionists following my lead) as a remedy for a broad range of illnesses that now dominate our health picture. Thus far, linseed oil taken alone seems more generally effective than fish oils alone, although combinations of linseed, fish, and evening primrose oils can sometimes provide the best effect. (We'll discuss this later.)

6. My work also shows a nutritional relation between the amount of dietary fiber, Omega-3 EFA, selenium, and other antioxidants in the diet and the intake of saturated fat, sugar, cholesterol, and "funny fats" formed by hydrogenation, for they all influence production of important regulatory fats discussed later. (Exercise and stress also play a role.) Since all these have been distorted in the modern diet, the result is a new kind of synergistic malnutrition. The Omega Program—the *first* complete supplement and dietary program—is specifically designed to correct this condition.

The reason linseed oil and its other dietary cofactors can help so many illnesses is that the major illnesses dominating modern societies—from mental illness and obesity to heart, bowel, and many other problems—are merely different expressions of an unrecognized nutritional disease. This new disease is a chemical variation of the classical B-vitamin deficiency diseases of pellagra and beriberi. These diseases all produce a wide array of seemingly different illnesses resulting from multiple modifications of the modern diet compared to the traditional evolutionary diet. Dietary modifications have adversely affected cooperating EFA and B vitamins to distort body regulatory processes, thus producing diverse illnesses, varying from person to person depending on genetic susceptibility. All this arises because modern multiple food modifications have never been adequately tested by health authorities for their collective effects.

When our national authorities recommend more fish and fiber to reduce the current epidemic of heart disease, they are still failing to state:

• That these recommendations are now necessary to correct a longstanding national dietary deficiency of Omega-3 EFA, fiber, vitamins, and other essential nutrients caused by untested modern food refining and selection patterns
• That the benefits of nonhydrogenated cold-climate plant food oils, which are high in Omega-3 EFA, are no less important than the benefits of fish oil supplementation
• That the benefits of returning to the traditional diet are not just limited to heart disease but extend to all the new diseases now dominating our health picture, ranging from obesity to cancer and mental illness. Many of these can be viewed collectively as an accelerated aging disease related to the B-vitamin-deficiency diseases pellagra and beriberi epidemic 50 to 100 years ago. The same food processing and selection patterns that removed the B vitamins at an earlier time now destroy our plant and fish sources of Omega-3 EFA, fiber, minerals, and vitamins, all of which interact to produce the regulatory fats controlling virtually every body function.

We often hear how Eskimos on traditional diets have less heart disease. They and other traditional societies also have lower incidences of arthritis, schizophrenia, irritable bowel syndrome—in fact, less of just about every modern malady. The bulk of illness today is not a medical problem, but one of life-style and nutrition, something you yourself must—and can—take charge of. .

Omega-3 EFA and cholesterol

Since there is a proven link between the consumption of saturated fat and cholesterol and the incidence of heart disease, it is a good idea to reduce the consumption of saturated fat and to increase your intake of polyunsaturated fats.

Cholesterol is not an ordinary fat but a fatlike steroid substance found in animal tissues. Cholesterol is an important part of nerve tissue and cell membranes. The gonads (sex glands) and adrenal glands use cholesterol to make certain hormones. The liver converts cholesterol into bile acids needed for food digestion and, at the same time, gets rid of excess cholesterol. A high blood cholesterol level is considered a risk factor for heart attack. People with diets high in saturated fats and cholesterol (an exact description of the average American diet) tend to have high blood cholesterol levels. These people usually are at greater risk for heart attack and other illnesses than people who eat low-fat, low-cholesterol diets.

In contrast to saturated fats, which have a tendency to increase blood cholesterol levels, monounsaturated and polyunsaturated fats lower blood cholesterol.

Omega-3 long-chained polyunsaturated fatty acids appear to change the balance of cholesterol in the blood. Omega-3 lowers the level of "bad guy" lipoproteins that clog arteries and raises the level of "good guy" lipoproteins that sweep cholesterol out of the blood vessels, where it tends to clog.

Eating one to two pounds of dark fish a week will help put enough Omega-3 lipids in your blood and thin your blood to keep your vascular system and many other functions in good working order. Or you can do about the same thing by taking supplements of nutritional linseed oil and increase consumption of unrefined northern cereals and beans.

My program is based on eating a high Omega-3 diet, carefully selecting the food you eat and the oils with which you prepare your foods. For those with overt illness, I add supplements of nutritional linseed oil (not the paint base), which will give you the extra Omega-3 EFA your body needs and help you look and feel better—and think more clearly than ever before. As a bonus, it may lengthen your life-span.

What do essential fatty acids (EFA) do in your body?

Let's review the fatty acid story. Plants and animals can make fats, starting from simple carbon compounds which they synthesize into fatty acids. The fatty acids we humans can make are known as "nonessential fatty acids," which means we don't have to get them from foods, since we can make them within our bodies. As already noted, the fatty acids we cannot make but need for good health are called "essential fatty acids" (EFA). Everyone needs them; too few of us get an adequate supply.

Polyunsaturated EFA make cell membranes more fluid and flexible. The cell inside the membrane is a tiny factory, taking in raw materials from the blood plasma and making and exporting a variety of products, among which are hormones. Everything going into and out of the cells has to pass through the membranes. Researchers have found that exchanges of materials between the inside and outside of the cell are more effective if there are sufficient essential fatty acids in the membranes. Insufficient EFA leave membranes stiff, unable to do their job. A deficiency of either or both Omega-3 or Omega-6 fatty acids causes a variety of disorders. Some of those recognized classically are:

- Skin problems—itching, flaking peeling, hair loss
- Headache—fatigue, restlessness, confusion, and general weakness
- Easy bruising, pain, inflammation, and swelling of joints
- Infertility, abortion, and kidney problems

Laboratory animals maintained on a diet lacking either of the two fatty acids developed skin problems (including rashes), were small in size, were usually susceptible to infections, developed fatty livers, and had defective reproductive systems and poorly developed brains.

Cholesterol: Villain or hero?

Normally, each molecule of cholesterol links with an EFA and travels smoothly through the bloodstream. When there is an EFA deficiency the cholesterol molecule is likely to become attached to a saturated fat molecule and end up as plaque—a fatty layer or protuberance stuck on the inside of an artery wall, creating a narrowing or obstacle where a clot can easily form and plug the artery.

Here is what happens when cholesterol molecules link with EFA:

- The body converts cholesterol to bile salts, which are needed to emulsify fats and make them digestible. This is also the only way the body can get rid of cholesterol.
- Male and female sex hormones and other steroid hormones are formed.
- Cell membranes in the skin are stabilized and strengthened.
- Skin cells are prevented from losing moisture (water), which would lead to dry skin and abnormal thirst.

OMEGA PROSTAGLANDINS

Over the past twenty years, medical interest in prostaglandins—extremely active biological substances, made from EFA, that regulate nearly every body function—has grown. Prostaglandins affect the cardiovascular system; stimulate the uterus to contract; regulate hormone activity, brain function, smooth muscle action, skin sensitivity, the immune system; and much more.

Prostaglandins are so vital to human life that in 1982, the Nobel prize in medicine went to three scientists who had studied more than a dozen prostaglandins, researching their potency and their role in directing almost every important function of the human body.

The EFA-prostaglandin connection

Prostaglandins are just EFA with a knot in their carbon chains. When EFA are added to the deficient modern human diet, the skin, heart, kidney, liver, and reproductive organs function better. Immunity to cancer and the ability to fight infections are improved. This is because the immune system and healing are in part regulated by the action of prostaglandins made from EFA.

Prostaglandins help to regulate the entire body. They help control:

- The inflammatory process
- The healing and repair process
- The immune system
- The neural circuits in the brain
- The cardiovascular system (including cholesterol levels and actions in the bloodstream)
- The digestive and reproductive systems
- Thermoregulation (your body thermostat, keeping your temperature at the proper level) and calorie loss

How prostaglandins affect your digestive system

The efficiency of the digestive tract from the esophagus to the rectum depends on peristaltic motion. The muscles of the gut churn the food in a kneading action, then propel the food in a wavelike motion through the system. All the muscles and sphincters of the digestive tract, with the exception of those in the anus, are involuntary.

The action of the involuntary muscles is stimulated by nerve centers called ganglia. Secretions, including those that protect and soothe the digestive tract, are also induced by the ganglia. Common digestive ailments—from gas to cramps and ulcers—can be caused by prostaglandin deficiencies or excess because the prostaglandins affect the function of the ganglia and body secretions.

Prostaglandins and healing

Prostaglandin imbalances can also lead to a loss of protective and healing abilities. For example, certain prostaglandins in the stomach govern the secretion of a protective stomach coating that prevents digestive acids from acting on the walls of the stomach. Without this coating the stomach would digest its own walls as well as food.

It is now suspected that ulcers develop when prostaglandin imbalance causes the safeguard to fail. The loss of similar defenses elsewhere in the digestive tract can also mean trouble; the kind and location depend to a great extent on inherited traits. Certain digestive tract disorders tend to run in families.

Omega-3 and prostaglandins—a key to improving digestive disorders

A majority of patients in my study who had long suffered gastrointestinal complaints, ranging from esophageal disorders to irritable bowel syndrome, showed substantial improvement and, in some cases, total remission when placed on high Omega-3 supplements (linseed oil) and the Omega Diet. They have maintained the improvements for over two years.

The more scientists learn about the function of prostaglandins, the more excited they are about the power and potential of these hormonelike chemicals, and the better they understand their origin and interaction with essential fatty acids.

Omega-3 and Omega-6 fatty acids each make a separate group of prostaglandins. For good health both are needed in the right ratio. That vital balance is hard to achieve because Omega-3 is often missing from modern diets.

A review of the role of prostaglandins

For all their importance, the role of the prostaglandins must not be overemphasized, for in addition to forming prostaglandins the EFA also

- Combine to form the lipids that comprise the cell membrane, regulating the fluidity of the membrane, which in turn controls the rate of manufacture of many cell membrane enzymes.
- Combine with cholesterol to control the transport of cholesterol to and from tissues and influence the formation of bile salts, which help to remove cholesterol from the body. Cholesterol combined with EFA also forms the steroid hormones, which have many regulatory functions of their own.

There are several classes of what may be called "active" or "regulatory" EFA. These collectively constitute a local tissue hormone system, which operates in most tissues of the body to regulate just about every body function. This local EFA hormonelike system contrasts with the classical hormones, which act widely throughout the body via the circulation to regulate activities at organ levels instead of at the tissue

Prostaglandins and Your Body

Prostaglandins regulate a host of body activities and functions. They:

- Cause pain or stop it
- Change pressure in the eye, joints, or blood vessels
- Induce labor, abortion, or menstrual cramps
- Regulate secretions and their viscosity
- Dilate or constrict blood vessels
- Increase or decrease collateral circulation
- Direct endocrine hormones to their target cells
- Regulate smooth muscle and autonomic reflexes: gastrointestinal, arterial, eye, ear, heart
- Control calcium and ion pumping in the cell
- Induce anaphylactic shock
- Prevent or cause peptic ulcer
- Control diuresis and salt retention
- Alter clot formation
- Regulate fever
- Affect tissue swelling
- Inhibit gastric secretions
- Shrink nasal mucous membranes
- Affect allergies and rheumatoid arthritis
- Regulate sunburn inflammation and complexion color
- Regulate nerve transmission
- Trigger cell division
- Control water evaporation from the skin
- Stimulate steroid production

The list seems endless—and it may be. Scientists are still discovering regulatory effects of the prostaglandins.

level. Finally, to these two regulatory systems—organ and tissue—must be added the familiar intracellular protein catalysts called "enzymes."

Altogether, there is a hierarchy of three regulatory systems, starting at the lowest level with the intracellular protein enzymes, going on to the fat-based tissue hormone regulators (the active EFA), and finally rising to the classical organ-level hormones. One of the main functions of the active EFA is to control the relations between the classical organ-level hormones and the intracellular enzymes.

Given the extensive regulatory role of the active EFA and the growing indications that both stress and exercise also work through them to produce their effects, we can begin to see why dietary disruption of EFA and EFA cofactors—vitamins, minerals, and fiber—can disrupt just about any body function and produce almost any disease, depending on the genetically determined susceptibility of different features of the EFA-based regulatory system.

Essential fatty acids help your brain function

The normal brain is about 60 percent fat. The scientists who have identified the complex fatty acids in the human brain found that the most abundant polyunsaturated fats are derivatives of the only two fats we must have in our diet—the Omega-3 and Omega-6 essential fatty acids. The Omega-3 EFA are even more abundant in the brain than the Omega-6. The brain's highly polyunsaturated Omega-3 and Omega-6 fats (we can call the former ultra-polyunsaturated fats) provide the fluidity needed for proper reception and transmission of impulses between the brain's cells. It's noteworthy that pregnant mice deprived of EFA gave birth to mice with small, underdeveloped brains.

The catastrophic disruption of dietary EFA

Three things have caused the reduction of EFA consumption: (1) a change in flour-milling technology, (2) a turn toward beef as a primary protein source, and (3) the introduction of hydrogenation of vegetable oils.

Not long after the turn of the century, when traditional diets were rapidly changing, the intake of EFA plummeted. Heavy steel roller milling replaced local stone-grinding of grains. The metal rollers produced white flour, which was inexpensive and had a long shelf life. Unfortunately, valuable vitamins, minerals, and fiber were in the "waste material" that was discarded. The leftovers also contained the embryo of the plant—the germ—a good source of vitamin E, Omega-3 and Omega-6 fatty acids, and other vitamins and minerals. But this germ was used for cattle feed, not for human consumption, except as a supplemental cereal, e.g., wheat germ.

With the growth of railroads, beef could be shipped to every part of the nation, and beefsteak soon became the most popular meat. Americans who had depended on local supplies of pork, fish, fowl, and game—relatively rich in Omega-3 and Omega-6—soon switched to beef, a poor source of Omega-3 and Omega-6 EFA and also very high in saturated fat. So American diets were further deprived of good sources of Omega-3 and Omega-6 EFA.

In addition, modern transportation allowed the use of southern foods and food oils in the north. These, too, have little Omega-3 (but plenty of Omega-6, as found in corn and corn oil, safflower oil, peanut oil, cottonseed oil, and so on). Warm-climate oils have displaced our traditional, indigenous cold-climate high Omega-3–containing northern oils, such as walnut, soy, chestnut, hazelnut, wheat germ, and linseed.

Modern technology is responsible for still another method of loss of Omega-3 and Omega-6. This is the process of hydrogenating oils. Hydrogen gas and a chemical catalyst are pumped under high pressure into an oil, forcing the hydrogen atoms to "saturate" the carbons in the oil, making it a poor source of EFA.

Why is this done? Because of rancidity, always a big enemy of food oils, especially with our new continental-scale feeding technology. Reducing rancidity means eliminating or decreasing spoilage, not only in oils and shortening but in any foods prepared with them. Hydrogenating an oil extends the shelf life. The more unsaturated (liquid) a fat is, the more vulnerable it is to the oxidation process that produces the rancidity. Omega-3 fatty acids are the special targets for hydrogenating because Omega-3 oils, the most unsaturated, become rancid most easily and quickly.

The trans-fatty acids are the bad guys

The chemical refining and hydrogenation of food oils that destroy EFA, especially the Omega-3, also create high levels of "funny fats"— trans-fatty acids or other isomeric fats. These "imposter" fatty acids behave like freeloaders, infiltrating cell membranes and stealing enzymes so that real fatty acids can't do their work. Trans-fatty acids actually increase the body's dietary EFA requirements rather than fulfill the body's needs, although they still provide calories.

Isomers and trans-fatty acids lodge in our muscles, liver, spleen, kidneys, adrenal glands, and heart. Less than a day after foods containing them are eaten by nursing mothers, trans-fatty acids show up in their milk. (The good news is that when trans-fatty acids are removed from the diet, their effects soon diminish.)

Polyunsaturated fats—introduced by popular demand

There has been a steady rise in the consumption of saturated fats in our country since the early 1900s. Was it just coincidence that this paralleled the rise in heart disease? By the 1950s, heart attacks were epidemic. Medical research identified saturated fats in food and cholesterol in arteries as the prime culprits. Unsaturated fats to the rescue! Doctors using polyunsaturated oils experimentally saw lowered cholesterol levels as well as lowered blood pressure in their patients. In fact, cardiac deaths declined, although a decrease in smoking in the general population probably helped, too.

A penitent cooking-oil industry soon changed its favorite product—solid, hydrogenated shortenings—to liquid oils. This was to provide a growing, nutritionally more aware market with oil that was polyunsaturated. New cooking oils and shortenings appeared on the market and were supported by advertising campaigns that featured the idea of good health. Many of the new oils had a higher percentage of Omega-6 EFA than before, but Omega-3 EFA was still missing.

In fact, calculations show that even today the net result of all these food and dietary manipulations has been to reduce the availability of the essential Omega-3 nutrient by a whopping 80 percent compared to traditional dietary levels. At the same time, the effects of the isomers produced by hydrogenation obstruct the path of between 20 and 40 percent of certain enzymes needed to utilize the EFA. The combined effect of all these EFA distortions is equivalent to reducing dietary availability by *far more than* 80 percent. And this is only the beginning of the problem.

Not all vegetable oils are the answer

The most popular food oils now are safflower, corn, sunflower, cottonseed, and peanut, all of which are low in cholesterol and high in Omega-6 EFA—but none contain more than traces of Omega-3. Soybean oil, normally a good source of Omega-3 as well as of Omega-6 EFA, seemed like the answer, but because of hydrogenation and the development of a soybean with little Omega-3, it has been a nutritional disappointment. Most diets are still deficient in Omega-3 EFA. (Coconut and palm kernel oils are high in saturated fats. Avoid them.)

Following the success of "natural" oils, new margarines with higher polyunsaturated oil contents were developed, and they were quickly endorsed by doctors and nutritionists. But the Omega-3 fatty acids in the new margarines were destroyed by "light hydrogenation," a process that also created artificial trans-fatty acids, or "funny fats," in the products.

GETTING THE OMEGA NUTRIENTS
YOU NEED

Omega-6 has been restored to many American diets via salad oils and margarine, but most still lack crucial Omega-3. Moreover, the presence in our tissues of trans-fatty acids that interfere with cell membrane function requires additional Omega-3 just to undo that damage.

With Omega-3 essential fatty acids stripped from our diets, do most of us get the nutrition we need? I don't think so. My calculations of national consumption and my pilot study involving forty-four people clearly support that fact. Although we human beings need very little Omega-3, we aren't getting even that small amount.

Linseed oil provides needed Omega-3

How much Omega-3 EFA do we need?

It is impossible to prescribe exactly either the amount of Omega-3 EFA any individual needs or the exact balance between Omega-3 and Omega-6 EFA that is needed. Human beings metabolize Omega-3 fatty acids differently. Each person is different, and at different times you need more or less of these important nutrients.

By evaluating various sources of data, I estimate that the average healthy person requires about 1 to 2 percent of his calories daily as Omega-3 EFA and about 6 to 8 percent as Omega-6 EFA. These figures can be regarded as the tentative recommended daily allowances for the two EFA families.

The best way to get the nutrition you need is from the food you eat. (The chapters in Part III provide menus and recipes for a complete high Omega-3 regimen.) Another way is to enhance your present diet—or even to boost the Omega-3 Diet—by taking nutritional EFA supplements just as one might take vitamin and mineral supplements.

Linseed oil is the ideal Omega-3 oil to take as a supplement. It is mild tasting, relatively inexpensive, and very safe. Most important, it works. Although the long-term effects of linseed oil supplements of Omega-3 EFA have not been determined, linseed oil has been used for centuries. It is a first cousin to the cod liver oil supplements of our youth.

Developing your own Omega-3 program

You must set out your own program dedicated to living a longer, better, and healthier life. What you'll need to know is the amount of Omega-3 EFA in each of the oils you use. That way you can select the foods that are nutritionally best for you. Here is a list of some of the unsaturated fats (oils). Note the amount of Omega-3 and Omega-6 EFA in each oil. Let this chart be your guide:

EFA Composition of Food Oils

Oil	Omega-3 percentage	Omega-6 percentage
Linseed oil	60	20
Salmon	30	20
Walnut	10	40
Wheat germ	10	40
Soybean	8	50

Oil	Omega-3 percentage	Omega-6 percentage
Safflower	1	58–75
Sunflower	1	20–72
Corn	1	40–57
Almond	1	14–44
Sesame	1	40
Avocado	1	10–40
Peanut	1	20–30
Apricot kernel	1	14–30
Olive	1	8–15
Coconut	1	2–3
Palm kernel	1	1–2

It's easy to see which oils are highest in Omega-3 EFA. You'll also notice that these high Omega-3 oils come from plants and animals that live in temperate or cold climates. Note that olive oil, which is high in monounsaturated fat and thus makes a good substitute for meat fat, does not contain much EFA.

Northern oils are best for high Omega-3. Most oils used today are from plants that grow in southern climates, or are northern oils that have been hydrogenated. The southern oils are very low in Omega-3; most have less than 1 percent. Cold-climate northern wheat, nuts, seeds, and beans contain more Omega-3 EFA than similar types of plants grown in a subtropical or tropical climate, such as non–cold-adapted wheat, corn,

---

The Potent Punch of Omega-3

If you're in good health, one teaspoon of linseed oil will supply the average daily requirements, approximately 2 grams of Omega-3 fatty acids, the minimum needed. This may appear too scant an amount to reverse a dietary deficiency, but essential nutrients are in a class by themselves when it comes to the power punch delivered by amounts smaller than a period on this page.

Many nutrients are very potent: A deficiency of only 2 milligrams (two-thousandths of a gram) of vitamin B_1 or three micrograms (three-millionths of a gram) of vitamin B_{12} can produce the killer diseases beriberi and pernicious anemia. Although Omega-3 oils do tend to become rancid, refrigeration, replacing air with an inert gas, or adding natural antioxidants such as vitamin E allow them to keep their full natural quota of Omega-3 EFA for many months.

sesame seed, lentils, and peanuts. Replace all your southern oils, nuts, and seeds with *nonhydrogenated* high Omega-3 products that come from northern cold climates. This is especially desirable if you live in a temperate climate or have ancestry that includes people who lived in temperate or cold climates.

Unless the human body gets its needed supply of both Omega-3 and Omega-6 fatty acids, it cannot make the needed prostaglandins and other regulatory EFA that are by-products of these fatty acids. Understanding the interaction between the two EFA families is necessary. Balance is what it's all about—balancing the EFA in our body and brain tissues, and balancing the production of prostaglandins and active EFA.

4
Fiber and Omega-3 Work Together

D*ietary fiber* is a generic term for plant materials that are not digestible. Fiber is the substance that gives plants structure and stability. Some fibers—cellulose, hemicellulose, and lignin—are not soluble in water but can absorb several times their weight in water. Cereal fibers are an example of this type. They exist in the outer husk of grains and are lost when the husk is removed during the modern milling process. Hydrophilic fibers—gums, mucilages, and pectin—are water soluble. Hydrophilic fiber, found in the nondigestible parts of fruits and vegetables, is present in varying amounts but is removed from fruit juices.

Fiber is not digestible but passes through the system. Nonhydrophilic, cereal fiber provides bulk to help eliminate body wastes and augments the action of the bacterial flora in the lower intestine. Hydrophilic fiber (fruit and vegetable fiber) helps reduce serum cholesterol by regulating secretion of bile salts, as mentioned earlier.

Recognition of the significance of the role of fiber has been the result of studies done in Africa by British investigators T. L. Cleave, D. P. Burkitt, N. S. Painter, and H. Trowell. Their studies suggest that lack of dietary fiber is a contributing factor in diseases of the bowel, such as colon cancer and appendicitis, as well as in coronary heart disease, obesity, and diabetes.

Why fiber is needed in your diet

While the Omega-3 and Omega-6 essential fatty acids control cholesterol in the blood, fiber acts to control cholesterol products in the digestive tract. Fiber increases fecal excretion of bile and acids from the bowel. Since bile acids are made in the body from cholesterol, existing cholesterol is then used to replace the lost bile acids. By helping to get cholesterol out of the body, fiber indirectly helps to lower cholesterol levels in the blood.

In addition, fiber may reduce the production of carcinogens from cholesterol. Fiber and EFA cooperate to lower serum cholesterol. Each can do it alone, but together they are more effective. Niacin—vitamin B_3—also brings down serum cholesterol, as do exercise and weight loss. These are prime examples of nutritional synergy, different diet elements with a similar effect that is geometrically increased when they are combined with each other.

The pioneering work of the British researchers was based on statistical evidence showing that the incidence of many illnesses increased after 1850, when steel roller milling of grains was introduced. These same illnesses also increase in non-Westernized societies soon after they become influenced by modernized food technology. My pilot study has shown, however, that modern milling destroys as much EFA as it does fiber, and it is clear that fiber and essential fatty acids are interrelated in many body functions.

To find out how much fiber you're eating, just fill out a photocopy of the chart below, placing a check next to the fiber food you've eaten today in the "Your Diet" column.

Rate Your Fiber Intake

Food	Amount in your diet	Fiber content (grams per serving)
Grains		
Bread (white)	1 slice	less than 1
Bread (whole-wheat)	1 slice	1–5
Cornbread	1 muffin	2
Graham crackers	2	1
Rye wafers	2	2
Cereals		
Bran flakes	⅔ cup	4
Corn flakes	1 cup	3
Grits	½ cup	8
Oats	½ cup	10
Puffed wheat	½ cup	6
Fruits		
Apples	1 medium	4
Bananas	1 medium	4
Blackberries	½ cup	5
Cranberries	½ cup	4
Grapefruit	½ medium	2
Grapes	12	3
Peaches	1 medium	4
Prunes	2 medium	4

Food	Amount in your diet	Fiber content (grams per serving)
Raspberries	½ medium	5
Strawberries	½ cup	3
Vegetables		
Broccoli	½ cup raw	2
Cabbage	½ cup cooked	4
Carrots	½ raw	2
Celery	½ cup chopped raw	2
Corn	½ cup cooked	5
Lentils	½ cup	8
Lettuce	1 cup	2
Peas	½ cup raw	7
Potatoes	½ cup	3
Spinach	½ cup cooked	7
Tomatoes	½ raw	2
Nuts		
Brazil nuts	½ cup	8
Peanuts	½ cup	9

Fiber deficiency causes other negative effects

In the course of converting wheat to white flour or converting corn or other grains to grits or groats, modern steel roller milling removes the grain's germ along with the fiber. Nutrients lost in refining are:

- B vitamins
- Selenium
- Minerals
- Fatty acids
- Vitamin E
- Fiber

All but the fiber are contained mainly in the germ.

My "Mixed Fiber Supplement" (see recipe in the box that follows) is designed to provide the optimum amount of daily fiber in your diet.

Studies now confirm that natural dietary fiber not only works to keep the digestive system in order, it also acts to:

- Keep fats and cholesterol in the blood at normal levels
- Normalize insulin production by keeping blood sugar at appropriate levels and reducing "rebound" hunger half an hour after eating
- Prevent cancer of the bowel
- Help offset any tendency to irritable bowel syndrome and diverticulitis

---

Recipe for Mixed Fiber Supplement
(I call this my "Fiber Cocktail" or "Fiber Appetizer.")

For a single serving:
   1 tablespoon miller's bran (available in health food stores)
   ¼ teaspoon psyllium seed powder (also available in health food stores)
   2 tablespoons yogurt (you can substitute low-sugar applesauce)
   ¼ teaspoon wheat germ (optional, but experiment with it)
   1–2 tablespoons water (to taste or consistency preferred)

   1. Combine all the ingredients in a wide-mouthed glass; mix together lightly. Wait about 5 minutes for the mixture to soften.
   2. Eat the mixture with a spoon; follow it with a glass of water.

NOTE: I find it convenient to mix a quantity of the fiber together and store it for use three times a day. (See page 106 for bulk recipe.)

Digestive disorders are only one manifestation of an interacting Omega-3 fiber deficiency. Others are hypertension, atherosclerosis, cancers, etc.

Fiber alone is not the answer

Fiber alone does not end the problems caused by deficiencies of Omega-3 essential fatty acids. While adding nutrient supplements such as selenium and vitamins E and C also augments recoveries, vitamins and minerals alone cannot do the job either. Many of my patients had been taking supplements for years—some in megadose amounts—and some had even added fiber to their diets. But they did not enjoy true health until Omega-3 essential fatty acids were added to the diet. The digestive ailments, along with many other chronic symptoms, respond to supplements of fiber best when Omega-3 EFA is also part of the diet.

Omega-3 is the nutritional key that can unlock total good health. It is the nutritional missing link needed to ensure the efficient working of many body systems.

5
The Seven Factors
That Affect Your Health

Two families of fatty acids, Omega-3 and Omega-6, act together as the principal players in the complex drama of today's nutrition. However, they are affected by other factors that also affect your health.

Factor 1: Genes—what you inherit

As with looks, genetically directed nutrition requirements and disease susceptibility can be inherited. A genetically weak enzyme system or an inclination toward poor absorption of certain nutrients can cause dietary requirements for B vitamins, minerals, antioxidants, fiber, or EFA to be far above normal.

Genetic variations also make some people susceptible to emotional strain, "Type A personality," or other types of restless and excitable behavior. In some people even minor irritation can cause the outpouring of steroids and other hormones, which raise the requirements for all nutrients. When there is a nutritional deficiency, the prostaglandins and the rest of the EFA-based regulatory system suffer. The results may include disease with the same disease striking several members of the same family because of genetic predisposition.

Factor 2: An EFA deficiency

An Omega-3 deficiency is usually the issue. This can be caused by a dietary deficiency, by an excessive Omega-6 intake disturbing the balance of Omega-3 to Omega-6 in the body, or by "funny fats." Any of these can block the ability of the body to use the EFA.

Factor 3: Vitamin/mineral/antioxidant deficiency

Deficiencies in B vitamins and minerals are common in a large part of our population, which gets most of its carbohydrates from refined flour and sugar. Vitamin B_6 is removed from refined cereal products and is not routinely added back as are vitamins B_1, B_2, and B_3. This deficiency hampers the EFA-prostaglandin system because B vitamins help process dietary EFA into active EFA.

There can also be a deficiency in trace minerals since they, too, are located in the grain's germ. The minerals that work as cofactors in enzymes and are involved in the processing of EFA include, among others, magnesium, zinc, copper, selenium, and cobalt. When deficiencies arise from a scarcity of antioxidants, namely vitamins pro-A, C, E, and selenium and the amino acids cysteine and methionine, the EFA are destroyed. This reduces the production of regulatory EFA and also produces toxic by-products.

Factor 4: Fiber deficiency

EFA and fiber work as cooperating controllers of fats and cholesterol. A lack of fiber creates a secondary deficiency of EFA by allowing EFA destruction in the gut. Additional essential fatty acids will be needed to counter the high blood cholesterol levels produced by a low-fiber diet.

Factor 5: Exercise deficiency

Evidence indicates that regular aerobic exercise provides important benefits in lipid (fat) metabolism, the immune system, and the cardiovascular system; there are psychological benefits in stress reduction, as well. In an experiment, a colony of primates on a high-fat (atherogenic) diet showed reduced artery plaque when allowed to exercise aerobically for one hour three times a week over a year.

Factor 6: Stress

Stress affects your body by bringing the steroid system, related to EFA-cholesterol metabolism, and EFA, into play. Stress increases the nutritional need for EFA-prostaglandins. Evidence in the pilot study showed that Omega-3 supplements in combination with fiber and vitamin supplements led to greater calm and emotional strength.

Factor 7: Antinutrients and toxicity

Prostaglandin formation and EFA utilization are inhibited by:

- Too much saturated fat in the diet
- Trans-fatty acids in the diet
- High intake of refined sugar and flour
- Caffeine, alcohol, and smoking
- Recreational drugs
- Careless monitoring of prescription drugs

- Environmental pollutants
- Stress increasing nutrient requirements

The dietary elements included in this list are not really nutrients, but antinutrients. They drain, supplant, or inhibit the actions of nutrients the body needs for proper functioning. One kind of antinutrient comes from shortening and margarine. The heating and reheating of commercial food oils—a common practice in restaurants and fast-food stores—converts some of the fatty acids to ring-type molecules known as "lactones." Large amounts of lactone may interfere with the natural enzyme plasmin, which breaks up blood clots in arteries. Moderate exercise can increase plasmin's clot-dissolving activity.

A Food Damage Report— Nutrient Depletion in Modern Times

The dietary components affecting the seven factors have all been distorted in the modern diet. Here is a summary of nutrient intake now compared to 100 years ago:

- Omega-3 is down 80 percent.
- B vitamins are estimated to be down to about 50 percent of the daily requirement.
- An estimated 20 percent of today's population lives primarily on fast food, soft drinks, and alcohol.
- Vitamin B_6 consumption may be low for nearly all of us because it is removed in grain milling and is not replaced.
- Vitamins B_1, B_2, B_3, and E have also been lost in food processing.
- Minerals are depleted in a similar way, including selenium (by more than 50 percent), which is an important antioxidant.
- Fiber is down 75 to 80 percent.
- Antinutrients have increased substantially in the modern diet—saturated fat, 100 percent; cholesterol, 50 percent; refined sugar, nearly 1,000 percent; salt, up to 500 percent; and "funny fat" isomers, 1,000 percent.

As if all this were not bad enough, food and dietary modifications do not merely add up to produce their damage; their effects multiply synergistically, because they interact together in the body to control the production of the regulatory EFA. Over the decades, this synergistic modern malnutrition sets the stage for illness, the type you get depending on your genetic susceptibility.

6

How Disease Develops

ntil the last ten to fifteen years, breast, colon, and prostate cancers and heart disease were rare in Japan. The traditional Japanese diet is low in saturated fats from beef and dairy products, low in hydrogenated fats from margarine and shortening, but very high in fiber and Omega-3 EFA and selenium from fatty fish such as mackerel and salmon. However, the Japanese living in the United States (and increasingly in Japan itself) share the same high rate of colon cancer, heart disease, and other illnesses of Americans. Similar statements hold for South Sea islanders and many other traditional cultures as their diet modernizes. The opposite can also be true.

THE DIET CONNECTION

Schizophrenia, like cancer and heart disease and diabetes, tends to appear in members of the same family. However, statistics show that all these diseases are rare in societies where traditional eating patterns include abundant amounts of fiber, minerals, vitamins, and both Omega-3 and Omega-6 families of essential fatty acids. Even in modern societies the incidence of these illnesses drops sharply when people abandon a diet of processed food and return to a traditional diet.

"The Norwegian notch"—a modernized nation goes traditional

The most clearly authenticated study occurred by chance in Norway during World War II. The incidence of schizophrenia, cancer, and heart disease doubled there after 1900, when Norwegians abandoned their traditional diet in favor of processed foods. Suddenly the incidence of all these illnesses declined a startling 40 percent. The decline exactly coincided with the years of privation during the German occupation of Norway.

What happened to the Norwegian diet during those terrible years? Because of the German occupation, hydrogenated oil and processed and

33

refined foods were scarce, forcing the Norwegians to revert to eating traditional foods. Beans, whole grains, and fish, once staples in the diet, again became daily fare. Scientists who studied the phenomenon, which I call the "Norwegian notch," found the 40 percent decrease in schizophrenia, heart disease, and cancer coincided with a 50 percent increase in the consumption of Omega-3 EFA in the wartime diet. Fiber consumption probably also increased, and we know margarine consumption fell very low. After the war, the Norwegians reverted to eating commercial and processed foods; heart disease and schizophrenia soon climbed back to the prewar levels. Nothing like this happened in the United States, Canada, and Australia, where the diet changed little during the war years.

The evidence of food damage

When traditional societies like the Japanese, South Sea islanders, and others transfer to the modernized diet, they develop the diseases associated with modernization in approximately a decade. Conversely, when modernized societies like the Norwegians revert to the traditional unprocessed diet, their modernization diseases noticeably diminish within a year or two. My own Food Damage Report (see page 32) is an analysis of the nutrient deficiencies of the 1980s and shows that major changes occur across a broad range of diet components, not just in Omega-6 EFA consumption. The statistics given do not reflect the problems brought on by chemical food additives.

Scientific evidence of the effect of this "modernization" has been obtained through experiments with monkeys who, when deprived specifically of Omega-3, develop similar problems. Appendix C includes a scientific article that gives technical details concerning specific Omega-3 EFA deficiency in other laboratory and human studies, all of which point to the same conclusion.

The anecdotal evidence includes the important case of a young girl suffering an abdominal gunshot wound that forced her to live for many months on total intravenous feeding. The nutritionists supplied the usual supposedly complete set of essential nutrients, using safflower oil (very low in Omega-3) as the sole source of EFA. Within two months the girl developed a large number of neurological problems—dimmed and blurred vision, staggering gait, changed reflexes, and other difficulties. Blood studies showed that she had a marked Omega-3 deficiency. Intravenous soy oil (high in Omega-3) was then substituted for the safflower oil in her i.v. feeding. She recovered in a few weeks as her Omega-3 blood levels returned to normal.

Although the forty-four-patient study is but a single study, it is important because of the completely controlled feeding conditions and the laboratory data that emerged. The data indicate that some acute, short-term human neurological problems may well be the result of a specific Omega-3 EFA deficiency.

In the study mentioned earlier involving the colony of infant capuchin monkeys, it took nearly two years for the monkeys to develop their symptoms when similarly deprived of Omega-3 EFA. To complete this story, you should be aware of a well-controlled study on two colonies of rats, both fed identically from before conception through the next generation. The only difference was that one colony was fed safflower oil as the sole source of EFA, the other soybean oil. It took until they were adults for the safflower-fed animals to show significantly lower maze-learning ability than the soy-fed animals. So the "brainier" the animal, the more dependent it becomes on Omega-3 EFA. This and other evidence leads me to call Omega-3 the "primate essential nutrient."

SCHIZOPHRENIA AND OTHER MENTAL DISORDERS

Mental problems start in brain fluids

The human brain is bathed by cerebrospinal fluid. In the fluids that wash schizophrenic brains, the concentration of certain prostaglandins formed from Omega-6 EFA is sometimes more than three times higher than in normal persons. This excess, which can trigger irritation and inflammation in all tissues, including brain tissue, can occur in the absence of the balancing influence of adequate Omega-3 EFA.

If a human being is deficient in needed Omega-3 EFA, megadoses of B vitamins may trigger the remaining Omega-3 into action. Although the effect is temporary, vitamin B appears to neutralize an imbalance of prostaglandins, a task usually accomplished by the missing Omega-3 fatty acids. Since the early work of Hoffer and others, orthomolecular clinicians have supplemented the diets of mentally distressed people with many vitamins and minerals, and have also recently begun adding linseed and fish oil to the dietary program.

Early emotional difficulty may indicate a need for Omega-3

Many schizophrenics go through periods of severe anxiety before they descend into complete psychosis. During that time they try to carry on with their lives, although they may feel increasingly fearful. The same progression from anxiety to psychosis takes place in vitamin-deficiency diseases. Is there a pattern? How does this happen?

It appears that schizophrenia is genetically influenced but triggered by environmental-dietary factors. The disease often appears during adolescence, a time of growth and hormonal changes that create especially heavy nutrient demands on every body function, and often a time of emotional stress and turmoil.

Besides subsisting on poor diets, many teenagers and young adults further deplete their nutrient supply by excessive dieting in the desperate effort to be fashionably slender. It's a difficult task to get enough Omega-3 in any diet today, and a badly planned diet makes the task more difficult.

For a vulnerable youngster with a family history of schizophrenia, obsessive dieting and further reduction of already inadequate amounts of Omega-3 may set the stage for the appearance of psychosis. If sent to a hospital, such patients again live on fiber-depleted, Omega-deficient, high saturated-fat hospital food, plus candy, soft drinks, and coffee (often bought from vending machines). Given the connection between condition and nutrition, there's reason to be skeptical of chances for improvement in the hospital.

The mental improvement noted in the mentally ill subjects of my study was mirrored in improvement of their physical condition and was a direct response to increase in Omega-3 levels in the body.

The types of mental disorders

The neurotransmitters of the brain, which regulate information transmission between nerve cells at synapses, are under the control of prostaglandins. Because of this, brain circuits are highly vulnerable to dietary distortions. Those afflicted can come down with any of a huge variety of different behavioral disorders:

- If motor circuits are most vulnerable, the individual gets ordinary motor epilepsy.
- If mood circuits are afflicted, one gets manic-depressive disorders, a kind of mood epilepsy.
- If emotion circuits are afflicted, one gets fear or anxiety attacks—neurosis, a kind of emotional epilepsy.
- If thought circuits are afflicted, one gets schizophrenia, a thought epilepsy.
- If defense circuits are afflicted, one gets either agoraphobia (a reactivation of primitive defense mechanisms, retreating back to the cave for cover) or a paranoid attack; both are defense epilepsies.

And so it goes through the list of psychiatric diagnoses.

CARDIOVASCULAR DISEASE

The contributing factors

A heart attack (blockage of coronary arteries) or a stroke (blockage of cerebral arteries) occurs if plaques filled with saturated fats and cholesterol form inside artery walls, where they may enlarge and block the passage of blood. This generally occurs in combination with additional triggers:

- An excess of low-density lipoprotein (LDL) cholesterol carriers in the blood. These carriers deposit cholesterol.
- Too few high-density lipoprotein (HDL) cholesterol carriers, which are needed to remove cholesterol from the blood
- Platelets in the blood that clump too quickly and stick to artery walls
- Thrombus (blood clot) formation in the arteries
- Decrease in the natural clot-dissolving factors
- Spasms of the arteries, which narrow the passageway still further
- Stressors burdening the heart, such as chronic high blood pressure, poor sodium control in the kidneys, poor circulation, or obesity

The EFA-prostaglandin link with heart disease

Only a disturbance in the EFA regulatory system can explain this complex set of heart-attack triggers. In angina pectoris, the muscle spasm squeezing the coronary arteries and causing pain through consequent oxygen deprivation is related to prostaglandin-controlled spasms in other tissues. For example:

- Muscular spasm of the esophagus causes choking.
- Spasm of the colon causes diarrhea.
- Spasm of the ocular muscle causes vision problems.
- Spasm of the blood vessels to the brain causes migraine.
- Spasm of the uterus causes menstrual cramps.
- Spasm of the fallopian tubes possibly causes endometriosis

. . . and so on.

The high Omega-3 fat diet of some people, such as the Greenland Eskimos' traditional diet of fatty fish, apparently protects against heart disease and cancer, and probably also against arthritis, diabetes, and other diseases.

CANCERS

A known dietary connection

Even conservative nutrition and cancer experts have acknowledged that many cancers are primarily linked to dietary factors and that breast, colon, and prostate cancer are especially correlated with high intake of saturated and unsaturated fat. However, these experts have not taken into consideration that EFA are not all the same: The Omega-3 fats are different from the others. By increasing Omega-3 intake one can get enhanced EFA benefits while reducing Omega-6 and in that way reducing total fat consumption.

Fiber and cancers

A lack of fiber in the diet not only raises blood cholesterol but also may be an important factor leading to the development of colon cancer. Ample fiber dilutes any potentially cancer-causing by-products of fat digestion in the bowel. Fiber also speeds the rate at which irritating substances travel through the digestive tract, so there is less time to affect the delicate tissue of the bowel. Generous amounts of fiber in the diet also encourage aerobic lactobacillus bacteria, which create a climate of resistance to infections and cancer.

Cancer and your immune system

A vigorous immune system is your best defense against all kinds of cancer. The millions of cell divisions that occur daily within your body often produce mutants. If your own immune system did not destroy these mutants, there would be many more cancers than there are today.

EFA and the prostaglandins are crucial to proper functioning of the immune system. Prostaglandins also affect the liver's efficiency in detoxifying cancer-causing substances. Anything that hampers the EFA-prostaglandin system results in weakening the immune system.

DIABETES MELLITUS

This disease was known in ancient times but is an increasingly common problem in this century. Diabetes is now among the leading causes of death from noninfectious disease in the United States. Two hormones from the pancreas—insulin and glucagon—cooperate to keep blood sugar (glucose) at an optimum level. When it is too high, the pancreas sends out insulin to force glucose into the cells. If blood sugar gets too low for energy needs, glucagon mobilizes glucose and sends it into the blood for additional energy.

In people who are predisposed to diabetes by heredity, eating purified sugar can eventually stress the insulin production mechanism. Hypoglycemia, or low blood sugar, may represent a phase of diabetes in which a hair-trigger response from the overworked pancreas sends out too much insulin.

Diabetes and prostaglandin action

Like all endocrine hormones, insulin and glucagon exert their control over the cells by stimulating production of the prostaglandins. In turn, the prostaglandins pass the message of the endocrine hormones to the cell. Therefore, an EFA or cofactor deficiency interfering with the prostaglandin mobilization can produce an effective insulin-resistant diabetes even though adequate insulin is produced. This insulin-resistant diabetes is the reverse of insulin-exhaustion diabetes.

Juvenile diabetes versus adult-onset diabetes

The most serious form of diabetes usually strikes in childhood and may arise from an attack by the immune system on the insulin-producing cells of the pancreas or the insulin receptors within the tissues. EFA deficiency can cause the immune system to turn against the body instead of defending it.

In the more common form of diabetes that appears later in life, insulin is usually sufficient but is not effective in getting the cells to take in the excess blood sugar, glucose. An EFA deficiency can cause this inability of insulin to accomplish its mission by not providing the prostaglandin action needed to translate insulin's message to the cells.

Some diabetics have trouble utilizing or processing the Omega-3 EFA. This brings up the possibility that one of the genetic problems in diabetes and other modernization diseases may be an inherited tendency to process the Omega-6 EFA in preference to processing the Omega-3 EFA.

Diabetes and fiber

Controlled clinical studies now indicate that dietary fiber can reduce insulin requirements. I think Omega-3 EFA supplements can do the same thing. Omega-3 and fiber supplements plus the full Omega regimen provide the correct first-line treatment for this, as for other symptomatic expressions of the modernization disease syndrome.

A fiber deficiency, coupled with Omega-3 EFA deficiency, magnifies all the blood sugar problems. Normally fiber acts as a buffer in the digestive tract. It slows the release of sugar into the bloodstream. Fiber-rich foods also normalize cholesterol metabolism and reduce the requirement for EFA. Without fiber, the refined starches and sugars in processed foods quickly create a big surge of blood glucose and an exhausting demand for insulin.

Fiber supplements or foods naturally high in fiber, such as beans and whole grains, can reduce the amount of insulin that some diabetics require. As in heart disease and cancer, the hereditary aspects of diabetes can be controlled.

Diabetes and eye problems

A common cause of blindness in severe diabetes is degeneration of the retina of the eye. Just in the past few years, it has been learned that docosahexaenoic acid (DHA), an Omega-3 fatty acid, is the most prominent polyunsaturated fat in the retina. If diabetics do not get enough Omega-3 EFA in their diet, this deficit could be a factor contributing to retinopathy. Ironically, chronically high blood sugar in diabetes blocks an enzyme that processes Omega-3 from food sources into DHA, thus making the effects of any Omega-3 deficiency worse.

All of this suggests that the linseed oil Omega-3 regimen or its fish oil version, both described later in this book, plus the standard Omega Diet may prevent or ameliorate diabetes and hypoglycemia.

OBESITY

Nutritionists and scientists have declared obesity to be a serious disease. Compared with normal people, the obese (people more than 20 percent overweight) tend to have:

- High blood pressure
- Elevated levels of cholesterol in the blood
- Non-insulin-dependent diabetes
- Cancers (colon, rectum, and prostate in men; gallbladder, breast, uterus, ovaries, and cervix in women)

. . . and a host of other problems.

Obesity itself isn't the cause of illness, with the cure merely a matter of reducing weight. Obesity is just one more modernization disease symptom, caused by a deficiency of EFA and its cofactors and antifactors. Modern synergistic malnutrition can also attack the appetite-controlling appestat in the brain as well as the heat-controlling, brown-fat calorie-burning thermogenic system, so you take in more and burn less. The resultant weight gain has been properly called "no fault fat."

Obesity, stress, and your genetic makeup

Once obesity becomes a problem, it compounds other stresses or genetic weak spots. The continually high circulating levels of insulin and fats that often develop in the obese individual can exacerbate any cardiovascular or blood sugar disorders.

To overcome obesity, one must switch from the diet producing the obesity to the standard Omega Diet, which ensures that Omega-3 EFA, fiber, selenium, and all other required nutrients are supplied while also reducing antinutrient sugars, funny fats, saturated fats, etc. Proper exercise is also vital.

IMMUNE DISORDERS

Immune disorders are rampant in modern societies. They cover a huge range of illnesses such as rheumatoid arthritis, lupus, possibly alopecia areata, food and airborne allergies, chronic infections, AIDS, such bowel disorders as irritable bowel syndrome, possibly Meniere's disease, and many others. As we noted earlier, cancers also involve some element of immune disorder. Dietary distortions of the EFA-based regulatory system, including the prostaglandins, are now known to contribute to—even prompt—breakdown of the immune system. Many of these disorders respond to the Omega regimen.

THE "MAGIC SHOTGUN" TREATMENT FOR DISEASE

Notice that most of the disease-producing mechanisms—cardiovascular, cancer, diabetes, obesity, immune, bowel, mental—are known to be activated by the B-vitamin deficiency diseases of pellagra and beriberi, so we must expect them to be similarly activated when dietary factors distort the EFA that the B vitamins process into the prostaglandins and other regulatory EFA.

Striking back at disease means hitting the triggering factors

Although a large deficiency in fiber, nutrients, or exercise or an excess of antinutrients and stress can cause illness, I think the cause of many diseases is the synergistic effect of all those factors in combination.

When illness strikes, it can produce secondary problems: First, an illness may reduce the individual's ability to deal with stress. Secondly, further stress then makes the problem worse. Anyone who is functioning in less than optimal physical health can often be helped by the improvement of any area that reduces body stress. Most people will benefit from:

- Mixed fiber in their diet (both cereal and hydrophilic)
- Megavitamin supplements added to the diet
- Aerobic exercise at least three times a week
- EFA supplements of Omega-3 essential fatty acids
- EFA antioxidant vitamins pro-A, C, E, and selenium
- Two fish meals a week
- Reducing saturated fat, margarine, sugar, cholesterol
- Reduction of any allergy triggering foods
- Stress-reducing techniques such as biofeedback, psychotherapy, or support groups
- Going on the Omega Diet and regimen.

These steps taken together act as a "magic shotgun" and can be far more effective in addressing health problems than any supposed medical "magic bullet."

7
Health Benefits for the Omega-3 Program Volunteers

The Omega-3 program is based on the theory that health is a birthright, not an accident. Like life itself, good health begins in individual cells. We all start our existence as a single-celled egg no larger than a speck of dust. Fertilized by a sperm cell, the egg divides, creating other cells, which divide again and differentiate until billions of cells form a new person.

The Omega-3 and Omega-6 fatty acids are the main structural parts of every membrane surrounding each cell. The conclusion is simple enough: A balanced intake of Omega-3 and Omega-6 fats is necessary for healthy cell membranes and for creating the prostaglandins and other regulators that run the cells. I repeat: I think nutrient starvation is responsible for many if not most diseases today, just as it was during the earlier nutritional epidemics of centuries past. Today's public is starved of Omega-3 EFA.

Forty-four cases and their health problems

There were some striking similarities in the ailments suffered by the subjects in my Omega-3 study.

- Ninety percent had dry skin dermatosis (flaking of the skin of the scalp, eyebrows, arms, legs, and hands; fissuring of skin on the fingers).
- Seventy-five percent suffered fatigue (although they often didn't recognize it until they achieved real stamina).
- Fifty percent had an immune disorder (food or airborne allergies, rheumatoid arthritis, and others).
- Forty-five percent had bursitis, tendonitis, or osteoarthritis.
- Many had headache, itching or burning skin sensations, and tinnitus (ringing in the ears).
- Irritability was common.
- A number of subjects suffered all of these symptoms—and more.

These problems plus the major illnesses accompanying them constitute a syndrome. Because most cases responded to the linseed oil regimen, the conclusion is that they had the modernization disease syndrome.

The subjects' dietary background

Two-thirds of the subjects in the study ate moderate amounts of vegetables, salads, and fruits; enjoyed at least one portion of meat a day; ate white rice and refined wheat; used butter, shortenings, mayonnaise, and sugar liberally. Bakery desserts, ice cream, and soft drinks were popular.

The other third of the patient-subjects followed the same general pattern but conscientiously adhered to a "low-cholesterol" diet. Margarine was substituted for butter; they ate lean cuts of meat, used nonfat dairy products, and used Omega-6 EFA polyunsaturated salad oils freely. Their health was not appreciably better than that of the first group.

THE HEALTH BENEFITS FROM OMEGA-3 SUPPLEMENTATION

Emotional stability

After using the Omega-3 linseed oil diet nearly every volunteer reported feeling less anxious and more tranquil, calmer and able to enjoy "peace of mind." Some of the severely mentally ill also showed remarkable improvement.

Relief from dry skin problems

Americans spend a fortune on products designed to combat rough, dry skin and dandruff. Interestingly, laboratory animals suffer dry skin and dandruff when they are fed a diet deficient in EFA.

The forty-four patients in my study were typical; most of their skin problems improved on the linseed oil Omega-3 regimen. Dry skin and dandruff disappeared, and related problems (e.g., sallow skin and lack of elasticity) usually cleared within three months. Two patients with serious skin-related problems also responded well.

Improvement in cases of bursitis and osteoarthritis

Twenty of the fourty-four subjects had arthritis or the related problems of bursitis or tendonitis. Many cases were mild, others were moderate, and some suffered constant discomfort to the point that they were unable to work or required hospitalization. Nearly all of those afflicted enjoyed amelioration of their symptoms of many years when placed on the Omega-3 Diet. (The arthritis and bursitis returned in several cases when we experimentally substituted safflower or corn oil for the linseed oil.)

I define remission of arthritis as the disappearance of chronic fatigue, swelling, stiffness, pain, tenderness, and motion-restriction. (There may still be a need for a few minutes' warmup on rising, as well as an *occasional* need for pain-killers.) On this basis approximately one-third, or six of the arthritics in the study, improved substantially. In nearly all cases, there was a large drop in the consumption of aspirin or other analgesic drugs.

Rheumatoid arthritis is a disease in which the immune system produces antibodies that attack the joints. Those who were not already severely crippled found that Omega-3 relieved the swelling and inflammation in the joints.

Fluid pressure and inflammation in joints and bursae are regulated by the prostaglandins, and certain prostaglandins can trigger inflammation. Normally, body tissues produce prostaglandins that promote a soothing environment. In laboratory experiments, these "good" prostaglandins have been shown to stop inflammatory arthritis in animals. The Omega-3 EFA keep good and bad prostaglandins in balance, keeping those causing inflammation in check.

Amelioration of immune disorders

Among the most impressive results of the study has been improvement of the immune system. When the defense system of the body functions improperly, an immune disease develops. The body's natural defenders—spleen cells, lymph nodes, antibodies, white blood cells, and others—lose their defensive power or even attack the body itself. Half of the forty-four people in the study had some kind of immune disorder. Food allergies are a sign of an immune disorder, and many subjects had food allergies.

Correction of these disorders included amelioration of food and airborne allergies, chronic infections, discoid lupus, rheumatoid arthritis (if not too advanced), alopecia areata, and a number of other disorders thought to be of immune origin.

Why does the immune system fail? The tissues and organs of the immune system are no different from the rest of the body—they also require adequate nutrition. The evidence from the study indicates that a dietary deficiency of Omega-3 fatty acids is an important factor in the rise of immune disorders. Stress and deficiencies of nutrients such as fiber and certain trace minerals and vitamins will also contribute to these problems. In addition, heredity has a great impact on the form the immune breakdown will take, for allergies and rheumatoid arthritis run in families. When the body's cells are lacking the super-polyunsaturated fatty acids and prostaglandins needed to perform their job as cell regulators, the immune system functions improperly.

Case Histories

• A two-year infection of the hair follicles in the nose—a sign of an inadequate immune system—afflicted a fifty-year-old patient. This virtually disappeared after six weeks on the linseed oil regime, in spite of long-term failure on conventional antibiotics and steroid treatment at a major university hospital.

• A thirty-five-year-old patient who suffered severe rheumatoid arthritis for ten years recovered, but when she stopped the linseed oil or took it at a lowered dosage, the arthritis repeatedly flared up again. After two years on the regimen, she still requires large doses of Omega-3, but she is currently pain-free.

• A thirty-year-old woman who had developed a hot, swollen, and painful joint on her ring finger took two tablespoons of linseed oil daily. Two weeks after starting the program, her problem was completely controlled.

• A fifty-year-old woman who suffered crippling rheumatoid arthritis for more than twenty-five years noticed that pain and stiffness in her hips were markedly reduced after just three weeks on the Omega-3 program. However, her severely crippled joints did not respond.

• Under my general guidance, several other physicians treated a number of rheumatoid arthritics, using supplements of linseed oil, and noted exceptionally encouraging results, even in severe, chronic cases.

Headache relief

For years, migraine headaches accompanied the menstrual periods of one of my patients. The painful attacks disappeared after three months on the linseed oil regimen. They recurred in a mild form only when the oil was withdrawn in the week before the onset of menstruation.

Experimental evidence suggests that excessive production of certain irritating prostaglandins may be responsible for migraine. Omega-3 EFA tends to correct this.

In addition to relief of true migraine, four study subjects habitually took two to four aspirin daily to relieve tension headache. The headaches disappeared without aspirin a few months after the linseed oil regimen began.

Urinary problems—cystitis and enlarged prostate

A study subject had endured the burning pain and urgency of cystitis for several years but reported relief two months after starting the linseed regimen. She is still problem-free.

Three middle-aged men had enlarged prostates, with difficulty and frequency in urination causing interruption of sleep over a period of about two years. All reported that the problems disappeared on the Omega regimen.

Reduced incidence of cardiovascular problems

Two patients who suffered angina pectoris upon exerting themselves reported complete disappearance of pain within a few months after starting the linseed oil regimen.

A woman reported a varicose vein and pain in one calf that hampered her walking even short distances. She applied linseed oil topically to her leg, following the course of the vein, and found relief. (CAUTION: Some people have reported redness or irritation of the skin after applying linseed oil to open or ulcerated areas.)

Patients with hypertension (high blood pressure) showed decreased blood pressure. Two of these subjects went from moderately high to normal blood pressure; others were able to reduce medication dosage used to moderate blood pressure when they took the linseed oil. Patients with abnormally low blood pressure had it raised to normal. This is evidence that the Omega-3 regimen can normalize blood pressure in either direction.

Relief from menopausal problems

Two women who participated in the study were relieved of uncomfortable menopausal symptoms. One woman had been a cheerful and lively person at the onset of menopause eight years prior to entering the program. After menopause she became depressed and anxious, beset with weeping spells and the inability to think clearly. While Premarin (a type of estrogen used in hormone replacement therapy) helped, the linseed oil regimen permitted her to stop the Premarin entirely after a few months. Her mood vastly improved, and a number of other uncomfortable symptoms—including severe hot flashes—diminished.

Relief from irritable bowel syndrome

A number of those on the program were seeking help for gastrointestinal complaints, especially "irritable bowel syndrome" (also known as spastic colon or mucous colitis). Symptoms include abdominal pain, distension, rumbling, constipation, or diarrhea. IBS is considered to be a "functional" disorder with a wide range of triggers; it is the most common disorder treated by gastroenterologists, accounting for about half of their practices. All who suffered from IBS found some relief on the Omega program.

Some other outcomes

Itching, burning, and formication (a crawling sensation on the skin) cleared up in those who suffered these symptoms (medically grouped under the term *paresthesia*). Again, the connection to an Omega-3 deficiency was unmistakable.

Benefits of the Omega Program

Biochemical Effect	Clinical Result
Normalizes the body's fatty acids	Smoother skin, shiny hair, soft hands; increased stamina, vitality, agility, and a zest for life
Normalizes and rebalances prostaglandins	Smoother muscle action; improvement of many other functions
Reduces appetite provocation	Eliminates bingeing or addictive need for food
Stabilizes insulin and blood sugar levels	Keeps stamina high for long periods
Strengthens the immune system	Avoids or overcomes food allergies; fights off some diseases more effectively
Increases fiber and aerobic bacteria	Promotes proper functioning of the digestive tract to avoid gas, constipation, and other disorders
Normalizes blood fats and lowers cholesterol	Stronger cardiovascular system; clear thinking
Corrects the body's thermogenic system (ability to burn off calories)	Burns off fat; increases cold-weather resistance; increases comfort
Brings enjoyment of total good health	Improved quality of life

An unexpected finding was that within three to four months after Omega-3 EFA supplementation, a number of subjects who had suffered from declining alcohol tolerance reported a return to normal. This indicates a relationship between Omega-3 deficiency and the lessened ability of the liver to detoxify alcohol, and it may be a significant factor in chronic alcoholism. (Alcoholics Anonymous, please take note.)

A number of the subjects reported greater tolerance for cold weather after Omega-3 supplementation. The Omega-3 EFA in linseed oil stimulates blood circulation and plays an important part in resetting the body's "thermostat," which directs food or stored fat to be burned for heat. The Omega-3 oils have a special role in cold climates, where their super-polyunsaturated character provides extra flexibility to plants, sea life, and people—even at below freezing temperatures. We shouldn't be surprised at this finding.

Finally, many of the subjects started the study feeling wan and looking gray. Their complexions improved in texture and color after they began taking Omega-3 supplements. (As the "look of health" is so important to everyone, we've taken the next chapter simply to discuss complexion and diet connections that are now evident to us.)

8

The Omega Complexion Connection

Beautiful complexions come in every shade—from creamy ivory or pinky peach to burnished black or glowing copper. At any age or with any color, smooth, velvety, unbroken, luminescent skin is lovely to look at and signals good health. However, lovely skin often evades us, and each year more than $10 billion are spent on over-the-counter cosmetic skin preparations and medical treatments. More than vanity is involved.

What Your Skin Does for You

Skin is a protective wrapping. Your skin is your shield against environmental attacks such as pollution. Besides packaging the outside of your body, skin protects your body by guarding and buffering against:

- Ultraviolet rays of the sun
- Bruises from trauma
- Invaders such as bacteria

Skin also has important mechanical functions that affect other organs:

- Natural cholesterol in the skin absorbs sunlight to make vitamin D.
- Sebaceous glands deep within the skin manufacture and secrete lubricants to prevent evaporation of moisture and body fluids.
- Sweat glands moisten and cool us with water and minerals secreted from the blood, thus acting as an important temperature regulating mechanism.

Through its nerve endings, the skin serves as our principal organ of touch, as well as allowing us to perceive heat, cold, pain, and other stimuli. Sometimes, whether we want it to or not, the skin reveals our innermost emotions, as when we blush, turn pale, or become covered with goose-bumps.

Your skin's structure

Your skin is the largest organ of your body. If an average sized person's skin were stretched out like a pelt (an awful thought), it would cover about 19 square feet in area. Skin varies in thickness from 0.2 millimeters to 0.3 millimeters—thinner than a hair—on the eyelids, to about 4 millimeters on the back or shoulders. Skin on the soles of the feet is thickest of all.

There are two main layers to the skin. The *epidermis* is at the surface; the *dermis* is underneath.

The epidermis is composed of several cell layers. It is formed through the activity of the *basal layer,* a single layer of cells that constantly divide, creating new cells. New cells migrate to the surface in about three or four weeks. As you age, the migration slows and the same cells remain on your skin's surface longer and longer. Older, less efficient cells lose moisture and elasticity, resulting in a dry slack surface.

The dermis is made up of connective tissue. It contains blood and lymph vessels as well as nerve endings, sebaceous glands, and hair follicles.

Under the dermis, the *hypodermis* connects the skin to the underlying muscles. Composed of loose connective tissue, it also serves as a fat-storage and insulating layer. The hair follicles are rooted in the hypodermis, and so are many of the sweat glands.

Hair follicles—tiny well-like pores—in the skin send hair out to the surface of the skin. Nails are also a specialized form of skin (related to horns, hoofs, and claws of animals and birds). The outer layer of the skin, the hair, and the nails are composed of keratin, a specialized protein.

Inside the cells of your skin

An immense network of nerve fibers, lymph vessels, and blood capillaries bring nutrients to the skin and removes waste from the tissues. Skin is composed of about 70 percent water, about 27 percent proteins, about 2 percent lipids, and 1 percent sugars. The lipids (oils) in the skin are oleic acid, sterol, and neutral fatty substances such as cholesterol, all of which keep skin smooth and glossy.

Every cell in the skin—just as in the rest of your body—is surrounded by a membrane made of essential fatty acids. The cell's efficiency and health depend largely on these membranes. When a serious EFA deficiency occurs, the flow of nutrients and waste in and out of the cells is impeded. Protein manufacture and other cellular activities are compromised because the cells can't work well when structural membranes are damaged.

Skin and Omega-3 EFA/prostaglandins

Prostaglandins are involved in the cellular activity leading to both inflammation and healing. Groups of prostaglandins formed from EFA can trigger either process. When an Omega-3 EFA deficiency occurs, too many inflammation-inciting prostaglandins and too few of the prostaglandins that promote healing are available.

EFA deficiency has long been known to lead to eczema in children and to make the skin water-permeable, leading to excessive thirst. Moreover, the very rapid healing of the skin of my Omega-3 study volunteers indicates both EFA groups are needed to maintain balance in the skin's prostaglandin functions.

Omega-3 EFA are important in regulating heat production (thermogenesis), fat distribution, growth of hair (fur in animals), and circulation of blood to the skin. All of these functions are related to adaptation to cold climate—a natural role for the cold-climate Omega-3 EFA produced by the food chain in response to cold weather. An EFA deficiency in humans is often evident via skin rashes and scaling eczema. Improvement in chronic skin disorders such as scaling, fissuring, persistent infections of the hair follicles—occurred only after the study subjects began the intake of linseed oil.

The general color and elasticity of the skin also greatly improved among my study subjects. However, too much of a good thing is not good. If you overdose on the oils or vitamins—especially vitamin A—your skin will again become dry.

SKIN CHANGES IN THE PILOT PROGRAM

On the basis of the results of my study, I now think many skin ailments qualify as symptoms of an Omega-3 fatty acid deficiency, especially in combination with the rest of modern malnutrition.

Skin in the pilot program

In addition to other health complaints that had prompted the forty-four volunteers to join the Omega-3 program, fully thirty-nine of them had chronic dry and scaling skin problems:

- Raw, cracked skin, fissuring, and eczema (acute or chronic rough, bumpy scales and crusty, oozing skin) of the hands; chapped, raw knuckles and heels; and heavy callus formation.
- Scaling of the skin on the scalp. Most subjects had nonstop dandruff that didn't respond fully to special shampoos or treatments.

- Scaling of the skin on shins and forearms and flaking of the skin of the outer ear canal was common.
- Seborrheic dermatitis, a skin condition that is recognized by its flaking red, patchy skin. It is evident in the form of dandruff of the eyebrows, with patchy eczema around the eyes, nose, or cheeks and ear canals.
- Phrynoderma (scaling and enlargement of the hair follicles), resulting in rough, prickly skin on the upper arms, elbows, thighs, and tips of the buttocks.
- Sun sensitivity. Poor tanning with rapid sunburning affected several subjects.
- Acne plagued three victims.
- Discoid lupus afflicted one volunteer. This is a skin version of disseminated lupus, producing severe hair loss, scarring, and sun sensitivity and is thought to be an immune disorder.
- Alopecia areata claimed one victim.

The group response to linseed oil supplements

When the Omega-3 pilot study volunteers were placed on the linseed oil Omega-3 regimen, most noticed a rapid and marked smoothing and moisturizing of the hands. Many saw positive results within a week. As the healing continued, elbows, heels, and other parts of the body became smooth and soft. Within six weeks of the program's start-up, there was unmistakable improvement or even total disappearance of dandruff and the flaky dry skin on shins and forearms.

Several subjects plagued by an unpleasant winter tingling of the skin following bathing or showering noticed that this reaction disappeared almost completely. Most exciting was the fact that skin texture, tone, and color improved—in one to four months—as did skin elasticity and firmness; even wrinkles were less pronounced.

Three cases of long-term adult acne cleared up and one of alopecia areata diminished. There was a partial return of hair in the case of discoid lupus, a noncancerous skin disease with reddish patches which can leave scars and sun sensitivity.

Alopecia areata reversed

When coin-sized patches of hair suddenly fall out, alopecia areata is often the diagnosis. The onset of this frightening situation is often connected with great stress. Although in many individuals the hair loss may spontaneously reverse within a few months, many victims do not respond to conventional medical treatment and the bald spots remain.

This condition appears to benefit from modest doses of selenium (10 micrograms of the yeast chelate), supplemental vitamins and minerals, and, above all, linseed oil over a period of six to twelve months. My afflicted patients took these supplements for about a year.

Four months after starting on linseed oil, wispy colorless "baby" hair appeared. After eight to nine months, the new hair began to take on adult pigmentation; after eighteen months, new hair was evident over all the patches.

Phrynoderma roughness made smooth

Phrynoderma, also called follicular keratosis, looks like "goose flesh," except phrynoderma doesn't vanish when the shivering stops. To check whether you may have this very common skin condition, run your hands over your upper outer arms and elbows, thighs, and buttocks. The skin should be perfectly smooth. You may have phrynoderma if any roughness you feel is caused by hard white "flecks" of dried skin within or on top of the hair follicles.

Nine of the ten cases in the pilot study cleared completely within a few months. Phrynoderma responded to linseed oil supplements.

Again, improvement appears to result from reversing an Omega-3 EFA deficiency. Within three weeks of starting on the Omega-3 Diet, with linseed oil supplements, the skin of the arms and thighs was smooth, and soon buttocks skin began to smooth as well.

Acne cleared up

Acne results from an overproduction of skin oil by enlarged oil glands. This condition often occurs at puberty, when there is a sudden increase in hormone activity. If the enlarged and overactive oil glands become clogged, oil and other trapped secretions become home for bacteria; blackheads and whiteheads form, and pimples become infected.

Three cases of acne in a single family improved solely on linseed oil. Other dramatic improvements were seen on a regimen of one to three capsules per day of Maxepa (a high Omega-3 fish oil supplement). All the patients affected by acne (age twenty-two to thirty-six) had previously tried every accepted treatment with only marginal benefit.

Today physicians treat severe cases of acne with retinoic acid, a derivative of vitamin A that has spectacular effects in reducing acne. However, retinoic acid can only be used under a physician's care. It produces very unpleasant side-effects, including severe skin damage, and it has also been linked to birth defects. The success of linseed oil as well as of this vitamin A derivative may be related to the fact that vitamin A and the essential fatty acids share a common metabolism. Before trying the risky retinoic acid treatment for acne problems, I recommend four to six months on the low-risk Omega program. Interestingly, some of the unpleasant effects of retinoic acid, such as drying of the lips and elevation of cholesterol and fats in the blood, are problems that were corrected by Omega-3 EFA. Some acne may respond best to a combination of the Omega-3 regimen with retinoic acid.

Discoid lupus symptoms improved

Discoid lupus is not well understood by medical science; it is probably an immune complex disease. The characteristic facial and upper body lesions resemble those found in the serious autoimmune disease systemic lupus erythematosus, but discoid lupus usually doesn't involve the whole system and is confined to symptomatic reddened, dried plaques of damaged skin.

All discoid lupus treatment is largely experimental. One patient in the study who had had a severe case for more than five years began to show improvement two weeks after starting the linseed oil. His dry, leathery hands softened at the same time. By two months his hands felt reasonably normal, and the painful fissuring had disappeared. For the first time, he could go out in the sun and actually tan normally. Most impressive was a growth of firmly rooted hair on about 40 percent of the scalp that had not been irreversibly scarred.

The positive reaction from linseed oil Omega-3 supplements was very clear: When the patient temporarily stopped taking the oil for only two weeks, his skin began to dry and facial lesions returned. These improved again when he resumed the oil supplements.

Eczema significantly reduced

Eczema is a nonspecific general term referring to itching and sometimes inflamed, scaling, oozing skin. It is a synonym for *dermatitis,* which means "inflammation of the skin." No one knows why some people suffer this hard-to-treat allergic condition, which in rare cases can last a lifetime. Eczema is often accompanied by hay fever or asthma. About 7 million people in the United States are afflicted.

Eczema was significantly relieved in more than half the study cases by following the Omega Diet regimen.

OMEGA NUTRITION
FOR YOUR SKIN HEALTH

The skin problems resulting from EFA-deficient diets—such as eczema, scales, plugged follicles, and hair loss—are similar to those seen when certain B vitamins are missing in the diet. For example, pellagra arises from a deficiency of the B vitamin niacin, and pellagra is also associated with eczema and dry skin problems. What do the B vitamins and essential fatty acids have in common that makes a deficiency of either or both produce skin problems?

The B-vitamin/EFA connection

One of the fundamental functions of B vitamins is to convert EFA into longer, more polyunsaturated fatty acids. (They also help to convert those into prostaglandins.) For example, DHA, one of the more polyunsaturated EFA, can be formed from alpha linolenic acid (ALA) only if B vitamins are available. When either the B vitamins or the EFA are deficient, similar skin problems occur.

Zinc, EFA, and the skin

Until recently, infants born with acrodermatitis enteropathica failed to grow normally and usually died in infancy. They suffered from an eczema-like skin rash, hair loss, and diarrhea. The disease is due to an inability to absorb the essential trace mineral zinc. Fortunately, a simple cure has been found: Treating such infants with high doses of supplemental zinc results in complete remission of the disease.

Researchers have noticed that hair loss and skin defects, among which abnormal skin permeability (leaky skin), inadequate healing of wounds, and immunity disorders, can arise from either EFA or zinc shortage in the diet.

The zinc/EFA connection resembles the B-vitamin/EFA connection. Like the B vitamins, the mineral zinc works in conjunction with cell enzymes that convert EFA into longer-chain fatty acids, which become prostaglandins. Many of the ailments induced by deficiency respond best when both zinc and EFA are introduced into the diet, either in foods or supplements. This is another example of the powerful synergy shown by the essential nutrients.

EFA help cholesterol do its job.

Cholesterol molecules, which attach themselves to EFA, become stabilizing parts of cell membranes in the skin and elsewhere in the body. In an EFA deficiency, cholesterol is forced to link up with saturated fat instead of EFA. The stabilizing effect disappears and weak, leaky cell membranes result. This defect creates abnormal permeability in the natural skin, allowing cell moisture to evaporate from the skin, causing dry skin and even constant thirst.

An Omega Skin-Improvement Program

The Omega regimen of foods and linseed oil supplements produced striking improvement in the skin of most study patients. Although good results were obtained initially on linseed oil alone, long-term improvement was reinforced by *adding* the following to the daily diet:

- Small supplements of the antioxidant vitamins pro-A, C, E, and selenium
- Trace minerals, particularly selenium, zinc, copper, and manganese
- A multivitamin-multimineral one RDA supplement
- 5,000 to 20,000 IU of vitamin A, beta carotene, and vitamin B_6
- A few capsules per day of linseed oil, Maxepa, and, in a small number of cases, evening primrose oil. (Experiment to find the amount that works best for you.)

Skin improvements included softer, smoother, firmer, seamless, flawless skin and thicker, fuller hair. I also saw improved skin tone and color and reduced sun sensitivity; there was some fading of age spots on the hands.

The Omega regimen provides a program of nutritional cosmetology— from the inside out. Results include an amazing cosmetic improvement in the skin and heightened skin color, plus a sheen and fullness of hair that contribute to a more youthful appearance.

9

The Omega Topical Skin-Care Program

(in collaboration with Regina Flesch, Ph.D.)

The first step is going on the Omega Diet regimen. The second is being sure you exercise for a half hour or more at least three times a week. (See chapter 18 for the Omega exercise program.)

Improve your skin from the inside and outside

Omega-3 oils—linseed, walnut, soy, and wheat germ—can improve your skin both from the inside out and from the outside in. Many cosmetology secrets are based on applying oils to the skin; many skin lotions are naturally high in Omega oils—an example is jojoba oil—and they often also include antioxidants such as vitamin E.

Selenium (an EFA-protecting antioxidant) is the active ingredient in many effective antidandruff preparations. Vitamin pro-A, vitamin C, vitamin E, and selenium, because of their cell-building antioxidant properties, have been advocated for reducing wrinkling and as general anti-aging agents.

The essentials of topical skin care are easy to follow and will take you only ten minutes in the morning and ten minutes in the evening. You will be keeping your skin renewed and youthful.

Slant board technique

Many people find that ten to fifteen minutes a day on a slant board each morning helps wake them up. It improves the blood circulation in the face. You can buy a slant board or simply hang your head over the side of the bed. Or you can put the seat pillows of your couch on the floor, resting your body on them and letting your head rest on the floor, with your legs up on the couch seat. Some people find that a large ironing board propped against a steady chair or sofa works very well as an improvised slant board. During this time you can practice facial exercises, if you wish.

A morning face-wash followed by application of vitamin E lotion mixture and twenty minutes on the slant board with your head lower than your heart gives a special glow to the skin and makes you look and feel your best. (NOTE: Never use the slant board directly after eating.)

Morning Makeup

1. Wash your face using a mild antibacterial soap such as Neutrogena.
2. Rinse your skin completely, but do not dry your face.
3. Immediately apply a thin film of sunscreen or a moisturizer with a sunscreen to your face and neck.
4. Apply a hypoallergenic foundation color containing sunscreen.
5. Complete your makeup by applying your regular makeup foundation.
6. Follow the foundation by patting your entire face and neck with water-dampened cotton. This will set your makeup for the day. Your skin will remain fresh all day.
7. Use cosmetic colors—blusher or eye shadows if you wish.
8. Use a lipstick or lip balm with a sunscreen for year-round protection.

Daytime Skin Care for Those Who Do Not Wear Makeup

1. Wash your face using a mild antibacterial soap such as Neutrogena.
2. Rinse your skin completely, but do not dry your face.
3. For men, if you shave in the morning, be sure that your beard is well softened with water and soap or cream before shaving.
4. Rinse your face completely; be sure all soap or shaving cream is rinsed away.
5. Immediately apply a thin film of sunscreen or a moisturizer with a sunscreen to your face and neck. (Make applying sunscreen a habit; UV rays age the skin and are linked with many types of skin cancer.)

Nighttime Care

1. Wash your face with a mild soap. Be sure to remove all makeup.
2. Rinse, but do not dry.
3. Apply moisturizing lotion such as Lubriderm, Neutroderm, or a cream with elastin, aloe vera, or jojoba oil to your moist skin.
4. Allow the skin to air-dry.

Facials

Twice weekly give yourself a facial:

1. Wash and rinse your face.

2. Mix the contents of one capsule of natural vitamin E in the palm of your hand with your moisturizing lotion or cream. Apply this rich unguent to your wet skin and let it dry a few minutes before going to bed. (This mixture can also be used in the morning as a moisturizer, following the application of the sunscreen.

3. Finish by rubbing any residual vitamin E over the back of your hands, especially if they are dry.

TIP: Apply pure vitamin E to nonoily blemishes and eczema for fast healing and even-toned skin.

Seven rules of skin care

1. Enjoy the Omega regimen diet.

2. Exercise regularly and reduce stress.

3. Use the daily cleanliness-lubrication-sunscreen routine.

4. Stop smoking. (Nicotine constricts the tiny capillaries that bring blood to the skin, which may speed breakdown of the skin's tissues and eventually contributes to wrinkles. Heavy smokers have a typical wrinkling pattern.)

5. Use alcohol in moderation, if at all. Alcohol reacts with vitamin B, and needed water is diverted to metabolize alcohol within the body.

6. Use sunscreens. Ultraviolet rays are known to weaken and age skin. Wear broad-brimmed hats. Use sunglasses—UV rays can affect the corneas of your eyes as well. NOTE: Some medications (antihypertensives) and some foods (lime, celery, carrots, and cinnamon) make some people sun-sensitive.

7. Omegafy your skin. Creams containing polyunsaturated oils such as aloe vera and jojoba oil and vitamin E may be especially good for skin.

10
Omega-3 Nutrition for Men, Women, and Children

Most men and about 60 percent of all women between the ages of twenty and sixty work outside the home. The entire family eats meals and snacks away from home. Fast food and convenience foods, which so many people rely on, are practical, but are they nutritious?

WOMEN'S SPECIAL NUTRITIONAL NEEDS

More than other areas of total health, sexual health reflects a complex interplay of hormones and organs that are affected by diet. Women have special nutritional needs. Menstruation, pregnancy, and menopause are body stressors that require adequate nutritional support. Many nutritional deficiencies are related to diseases common in women—anemia, breast cancer, osteoporosis, migraine headache, and premenstrual syndrome. And, of course, a woman's health during pregnancy determines the health of her children. Three women in the pilot study who had suffered menstrual irregularity for many years all became "regular." In all cases, menopausal anxiety diminished and vaginal secretions improved. One woman previously without periods became pregnant, while many other health problems, such as arthritis and bursitis, improved when the subjects took linseed oil supplements and went on the Omega program.

Premenstrual syndrome (PMS)

PMS is a pattern of discomforts rather than a single problem. It is most likely to become severe in women who have suffered a hormonal change or who are between the ages of thirty and forty-five. Many women who have PMS also have irregular menstrual cycles. The syndrome includes some or all of the following just before the period starts:

- Nervous tension, mood swings, anxiety, crying, and anger
- Breast pain or tenderness

61

- Fatigue, dizziness, forgetfulness, headache
- Insomnia
- Food cravings, especially for sweet or salty foods

Although the exact cause of PMS is not known, it could be triggered by abnormal swings in hormone levels, prostaglandin imbalances, and/or an imbalance in the brain's neurotransmitter chemicals. All of these features are closely linked.

Supplements used in PMS therapy

PMS was once dismissed by physicians, but we now know it is real and treatable. Here are the vitamin and mineral supplements most often prescribed for this condition:

Vitamins: Vitamins C and E; vitamin B_6 is also often recommended.
Minerals: Calcium is a necessary cofactor in many metabolic functions; it influences the transmission of nerve impulses and activates enzyme reactions and hormone secretions.

Magnesium, chromium, and cobalt help to normalize glucose and reduce cravings. (Magnesium is present in chocolate, which may account for the craving for chocolate so common in PMS.)

Zinc is a cofactor that helps healing.

Omega-3 supplements of linseed oil or fish oils can also be helpful in avoiding or ameliorating PMS. Polyunsaturated fatty acids are components in every cell in the body; they are a key to determining the biological properties of cells. EFA also form prostaglandins and control many body functions dependent on EFA/prostaglandins.

Advice for fighting PMS

- Keep your weight normal; estrogen production is triggered by excess body fat.
- Increase the amount of complex carbohydrates in your diet.
- Get fiber into your diet.
- Restrict sweets and sugars. Candy or cakes can lead to mood swings.
- Eat small meals; keep your blood sugar and energy at a constant level.
- Limit salt intake to avoid water retention.
- Get regular aerobic exercise.
- Above all, get on the Omega program.

Menstrual cramps and how to fight them

An excess of Omega-6 prostaglandins is the major culprit in dysmenor-rhea, or painful menstrual cramps. The cramping of the lower abdomen, often accompanied by lower back pain and leg aches, can be severe enough to make many women uncomfortable for several days each month. The drugs that work best are those that interfere with the body's synthesis of the prostaglandins that cause the painful contractions. Unfortunately, these same drugs also hinder production of prostaglandins that relax muscles.

The Omega Diet offers a natural way to lower production of the offending prostaglandins without interfering with the body's ability to make good, relaxing ones. The soothing, muscle-relaxing prostaglandins are made when the Omega regimen of diet and exercise is followed. Following general suggestions for PMS will help. Additionally, because supplements of linseed and/or fish oils prevent overproduction of the prostaglandins that cause painful uterine contractions, these oils should be taken regularly one week before as well as during each menstrual period.

Help for infertility and vaginal problems

One of the causes of human female infertility is a thickening of cervical mucus; another is the potential spermicidal action of some vaginal secretions. An EFA deficiency interferes with normal secretions by tissues and glands. In animal studies, adding both Omega-3 and Omega-6 fats to the diet produced an increase in fertility—greater than can be achieved through pure Omega-3 or pure Omega-6 supplements alone. The Omegas

---

LInseed Oil Supplements
Lead to Baby's Birth

M., a thirty-eight-year-old mother of five-year-old Clomid-induced twins, had not had a normal period for ten years; she relied on drugs to regularize her menstrual cycle. She also suffered from arthritis and other health problems, including dry skin. When M. started Omega-3 supplements in the search for arthritis relief, she had some surprising results. She spontaneously started menstruating again; in fact, she soon became pregnant. At the insistence of her obstetrician, M. stopped the linseed oil supplements. Soon the dry skin, which had disappeared when she took Omega-3 supplements, returned. M. returned to taking one or two tablespoons of linseed oil daily and gave birth to a healthy baby, our first linseed oil baby.

work together, making secretions more fluid and less gummy and making body secretions a hospitable environment for sperm. In addition, amenorrhea and irregular periods can be regularized by the Omega program.

Linseed oil and/or fish oils, together with vitamin E and selenium supplements can be useful in increasing both female and male fertility.

Vaginal secretions after menopause

After menopause, a lack of vaginal lubrication and thinning of vaginal tissues caused by dwindling estrogenic hormones bother many women. Scant lubrication can produce such symptoms as vaginal dryness, itching, irritation, and painful sexual intercourse. These symptoms are often treated with vaginal hormone creams and estrogen replacement therapy (ERT). Inadequate vaginal lubrication is avoidable to some extent—when the Omega balance is right.

Consider the response in two postmenopausal subjects participating in my study. They reported an increase in vaginal secretions soon after starting linseed oil supplements. After only a few months on high Omega-3 containing linseed oil, the annoying, painful problem of inadequate vaginal secretions was greatly relieved.

MALE FERTILITY AND
ESSENTIAL FATTY ACIDS

Many researchers are concerned that male fertility and sperm count may have declined significantly in the past few decades. A dietary deficiency of Omega-6 EFA was rare in my pilot study subjects, but Omega-3 deficiency was common, and reproduction problems were also common. An essential fatty acid deficiency and a deficiency of the EFA antioxidant nutrients vitamins pro-A, C, E, and selenium, which protect the EFA in body tissues, are known to be a major cause of infertility in animals. Is it possible that the same is true for humans?

Male virility and food

The testes, the sex glands of male mammals—including men—normally contain a great concentration of docosahexaenoic acid (DHA), an Omega-3 fatty acid. (Prostaglandins were first discovered in the prostate gland, hence the name.) Human beings can manufacture DHA in their bodies from parent Omega-3 alpha linolenic acid or get DHA from fats and oils in fish and shellfish by eating those foods. With an undersupply of DHA, the male sexual system is left in less than ideal working order. Several men in the Omega-3 study who took linseed oil supplements reported an increased sex drive.

Folklore citing oysters as "virility food" may have a basis in fact, since oysters contain zinc and Omega-3, which are essential for male reproductive organ health. Many species of oysters and other shellfish, which are otherwise low in fat, are rich in Omega-3 EPA and DHA.

Prostatic hypertrophy

When the male prostate gland enlarges and presses on the urethra, the condition is known as prostatic hypertrophy. One of the symptoms is a loss of sound sleep, because victims wake several times a night to urinate. It can also interfere with sexual potency. Today, a swollen prostate is so common in men over forty that it is considered an unavoidable, irreversible symptom of middle age.

Is prostatic hypertrophy truly "natural" as men get older or just another disorder caused by modern malnutrition? The amazing recoveries by three men in the study who took Omega-3 oil supplements indicate the latter.

I put the men who suffered from prostate problems on the Omega regimen, with excellent results in each case. Two men in their fifties who suffered prostatic hypertrophy recovered completely from typical benign swelling of the prostrate gland. A third man was a physician who treated himself using my suggestions published in the professional literature; he felt linseed oil actually saved him from imminent prostate surgery.

Supplemental zinc has also been helpful in treating problems affecting male sex organs. Zinc acts in conjunction with essential fatty acids in the body.

OMEGA PRENATAL CARE

Creating a body healthy enough to conceive and bear a child is an important responsibility. The effects of alcohol, drugs, nicotine, caffeine, and stress during pregnancy have been widely studied in recent years. Clearly, it is best to avoid all of these non-nutritive factors. However, insufficient emphasis is given to preconception nutrition, especially to the nutritional missing link—the Omega-3 EFA.

Eating to make healthy babies

To improve your chances of giving birth to a healthy, happy baby, you should follow certain guidelines (after discussing them with your physician) when planning pregnancy:

- Both the prospective mother and father should be on the Standard Omega Diet for at least six months before conception.

- Before and after conception, choose foods that supply an abundance of Omega-3 and Omega-6 fatty acids. These foods include temperate and cold-climate fish such as salmon or bluefish, northern nuts (such as walnuts), grains such as winter wheat, northern oil (such as linseed).
- During pregnancy, the woman should consume a high-EFA, high-fiber, high-nutrient diet. Take a one-a-day multivitamin and multimineral supplements including selenium, manganese, calcium, zinc, and folic acid.
- The woman should increase caloric and essential nutrient intake during pregnancy to about 10 to 15 percent above normal level. (To find your normal intake level, see page 171.) A weight gain of close to three pounds a month, for a total of twenty-five to thirty-five pounds, is recommended for women of average build.
- Women should never attempt to lose weight during pregnancy.

Prenatal Development and the Immune System

The immune system is programmed during intrauterine development and in the early months after birth. Essential fatty acids are needed for a healthy immune system. Malnutrition in the critical prenatal period, including an Omega-3 fatty acid deficiency, can make the developing child vulnerable to both mental and physical illnesses related to a weakened immune system and other problems.

The developing brain

In 1968, Swedish scientist Lars Svennerholm showed that DHA, the super-polyunsaturated Omega-3, was the major unsaturated fat in the brain and that Omega-6 arachidonic acid was second in prominence.

Long-chained, polyunsaturated derivatives of dietary EFA are indispensable for the brain and nervous system of both a prospective mother and her developing child. DHA and arachidonic acid are preferentially taken by the fetus for the fetal brain. This is especially true during the last trimester of pregnancy, when there is tremendous growth in fetal brain tissue. (NOTE: DHA and arachidonic acid are also found in very high amounts in the retina of the eye, the thymus gland, and the testes.)

Like an adult human, the unborn child can make fat, but also like an adult, it cannot make essential fatty acids. The fetus must get EFA from the mother, who must get them from her food or from EFA supplies in her own tissues. A serious deficiency of EFA in the mother means the fetus is unable to obtain the EFA needed for brain function. Since the fetus and infant even have trouble making EPA and DHA from linolenic acid, fish and fish oil supplements become especially important during pregnancy and early childhood. Remember cod liver oil?

Scientists agree on nutritional needs for developing brain cells

In 1983, Italian scientists C. Galli and A. Socini, discussing dietary lipids in prenatal development, wrote: "The central nervous system in man undergoes an accelerated growth phase during the last stage of pregnancy and during the first month of extrauterine life and requires a high supply of EFA for structural expansion; it follows that intrauterine malnutrition may produce a low-birth-weight infant, possibly suffering significant, perhaps irreversible developmental damage to the brain."

Scientists agree. Much of the brain cell division needed for normal development occurs during foetal growth. Since brain cells and neural pathways have a high content of essential fatty acids, ultimately derived from the diet, it comes as no surprise to learn that "experimental depletion of these long-chained polyunsaturated fatty acids (PUFA) is associated with functional distortions and high perinatal mortality."

The findings are clear. Unfortunately, in America pregnant and nursing mothers are routinely reassured that all EFA needs are amply filled by salad oils such as corn or safflower oil. This just isn't so. Pregnant women and new mothers need supplements of oils high in Omega-3 EFA.

11

The Omega Factor in Breast-Feeding and Formula Feeding

nless there is the most compelling reason for not breast-feeding, mothers should breast-feed their infants for at least six months after birth, preferably for up to two years.

Breast-feeding is best

There is no comparable substitute for the remarkable mix of nutrients and immunity-boosting factors provided by mother's milk, as long as the mother is eating properly. A well-nourished nursing mother provides her infant with a perfect blend of essential fatty acids and their long-chained derivatives, assuring the fast-growing brain and body tissues a rich supply. Mother's milk also supplies important antibodies not present in cow's milk or in artificial formula.

The premature infant especially needs breast milk for its immature system. I know several mothers of "preemies" who, unable to nurse, hired wet nurses or secured human milk for their babies. The results were well worth the trouble. The infant on formula is not usually as well nourished as the breast-fed infant. Much-needed long-chain fats are present only in trace amounts in cow's milk formulas. Here is a nutritive comparison:

- Breast milk may have five times more arachidonic acid and two and a half times more EPA than formula.
- Breast milk may have thirty times more DHA than formula.
- Compared with mother's milk, formulas are also low in selenium and biotin.

The unborn child avidly absorbs arachidonic acid, DHA, and EPA derived from the foods consumed by the mother. The newborn baby does the same with these fatty acids in breast milk. If a pregnant woman's diet includes the same amount of Omega-3 EFA as she can get in one table-spoon of linseed oil—even if her diet doesn't provide adequate arachidonic acid, DHA, and EPA—her cell enzymes can make the needed arachidonic acid from linoleic, and DHA and EPA from alpha linolenic. If a mother breast-feeds, her diet should include the equivalent of one or more tablespoons of linseed oil. In addition, she should take a fish oil supplement— about one to two teaspoons of cod liver oil.

Another breast-feeding plus

During nursing, 10 to 15 percent more calories and nutrients are required than during pregnancy. There's another plus for nursing mothers: Women who breast-feed often return to their prepregnancy weight more rapidly than do mothers who bottle feed their infants. Not only does nursing burn up 500 to 1,500 calories a day, but nursing stimulates uterine contraction and in that way encourages the uterus to return to its normal size and shape.

How to make your formula better

Today's formulas are improved in many respects, but unless nonhydrogenated soybean oil or, even better, cod liver oil is in the formula, most contain too little Omega-3 EFA. Even when soybean oil is included for its linoleic content, manufacturers generally use partially hydrogenated oils that do not have Omega-3 alpha-linolenic. The exceptions are hypoallergenic infant formulas put out by Syntex, Neo-Mull-Soy liquid, and Loma Linda's Soylac, which use nonhydrogenated soybean oil as additions to the cow's milk base.

When not to breast-feed

Mother's milk can have drawbacks. Here are two counter-indications for breast feeding:

- If the mother's diet is full of saturated fats such as meat fat
- If the mother's diet is lacking in nutrients such as Omega-3, selenium, and biotin. The absence of certain nutrients in the mother's milk would be an indication of a lack in the mother's diet.

In either of these situations, the mother should go on the Omega program.

Sadly, the breast milk of many mothers in our country reflects the high trans-fatty acid and low Omega-3 content in the average diet. American mothers produce milk that often has only one-fifth to one-tenth of the Omega-3 content of the milk that well-nourished, nut-eating Nigerian mothers provide their infants.

The need for long-chain fatty acids in formulas

New research on infant feeding has uncovered the answer to a pressing question: Can unborn or very young infants, including premature babies, readily convert EFA into long-chain fatty acids in the large amounts needed in the developing organs, such as the eyes and the brain? Several studies suggest that much of the converting is done for the fetus by the mother's enzymes and by enzymes in the placenta. Infants may not be able to convert the EFA until several weeks after birth.

Not too many years ago, many infants developed eczema due to formulas low in EFA. Today most infant formulas contain ample (some researchers say excessive) amounts of Omega-6 linoleic acid. A few formula manufacturers add some Omega-3 alpha linolenic to their formulas, but in most cases I believe it is too little for any positive nutritional effect.

Infant formulas should include fish oils such as cod liver oil. Since none of those commercially available have these oils added, you must add your own to the tune of about five to ten drops to each day's formula supply. During the 1940s, cod liver oil was routinely given to infants by medicine dropper. Later that practice was abandoned—but it should be revived. Fish oils provide a full complement of long-chain Omega-3 and Omega-6 fatty acids. These may be crucial for young infants and "preemies" on formula. I recommend returning to the practice of adding ten drops of cod liver oil to the baby's formula or giving it orally from a medicine dropper. (For more on this topic, see chapter 22.)

Human milk is best for babies. It is preferable to the new "improved" formulas. Pediatrician Lendon Smith finds eczema to be far less a problem in breast-fed than in bottle-fed babies. Someday consumer pressure may spur the development of a sensible, safe way to maintain the Omega-3 content of products while avoiding the economic and health risks of rancidity. A feasible solution will be found once a big market exists for nutritionally superior products.

OMEGA DEFICIENCY IN EARLY CHILDHOOD

The effects of EFA deficiency in pregnancy and infancy can show up in any number of ways. For example, extended colic in infants can be a juvenile form of the adult irritable bowel syndrome. Many disorders of the digestive system originate from the disproportionate production of Omega-6 prostaglandins that are not balanced by sufficient Omega-3 EFA. Since prostaglandins are produced locally in all our cells and tissues, the same sort of inflammatory prostaglandins can be associated with irritation anywhere—not just in the nerves of the digestive tract but also in the kidneys, bronchial passages, joints, and even in the brain.

The Omega baby and toddler diet

When your baby starts on solid food, you should enrich the child's diet by preparing or selecting prepared baby foods that are:

- Low in sugar
- Free of any hydrogenated oils (read labels)
- High in nonhydrogenated Omega oils such as soybean and walnut
- Easy to chew
- High in fiber (try fiber cocktail, cook vegetables lightly, use stone ground cereals)

Adequate fiber intake is important not only for a child's general health but also for bowel training, because sufficient dietary fiber prevents painful constipation. Pureeing adult food in the Omega-3 Diet makes it easy for baby to join the family in savoring a wide variety of wholesome, traditional dishes. (See Part III of this book.)

Sudden infant death syndrome (SIDS) may respond to Omega-3

Sudden infant death syndrome, or "crib death," appears to have some of the same features as a disorder involving the esophagus and the swallowing reflex suffered by several Omega-3 deficient adults in my study. The adults would suddenly be unable to breathe, often to the point of almost suffocating. Studies of "crib death" show that:

- A high proportion of SIDS infants were on formulas that lacked Omega-3 fatty acids.
- Formulas often contain very low levels of biotin, the vitamin involved in EFA metabolism (cow's milk is low in biotin).
- Several autopsies showed that the babies who died had low circulating levels of vitamin E and selenium, which are needed to protect EFA from oxidation.

Low levels of Omega-3 EFA, biotin, and selenium, combined with high levels of trans-fatty acids in infant formula result in infant malnutrition. Malnutrition doesn't always cause obviously slow growth or poor weight gain. It can be far more insidious, affecting all aspects of health and behavior in infancy, childhood, and later life. Many symptoms are less obvious initially than low growth rates or below-normal weight.

A treatment for hyperactive children

A 1979 study claims that from 25 to 50 percent of hyperactive children become delinquent or develop other problems requiring institutionalization on approaching or reaching adulthood. In 1982, a pediatrics researcher reported that generalized malnutrition can affect later emotional and social development. Clearly, one of the signs of malnutrition can be hyperactive behavior.

A support group for English parents of hyperactive children reports that affected children suffer from:

Food sensitivity	Infantile colic	Eczema	Ear infections
Runny noses	Chest infections	Asthma	

These problems look like just another variant of the modernization disease syndrome (MDS). Parents in the group speculate that these ailments arise from a weakened immune system. Hyperactive or not, English children—just as their American counterparts—often suffer an Omega-3 dietary deficiency plus an overload of trans-fatty acids. For example, phrynoderma is very common in English school children. A low or inadequate production of specific prostaglandins may be partly responsible.

Supplements of oil of evening primrose were helpful in about half of a group of twenty-five hyperactive children who were given the supplement. Evening primrose oil is high in gamma linolenic, an Omega-6 fatty acid. (This same fatty acid is also found in breast milk.) Gamma linolenic can be converted in the body to soothing prostaglandins that counter the inflammatory prostaglandins that often trigger emotional storms as well as physical upsets in children. Besides oil of evening primrose, it makes sense to supply children with linseed and/or fish oils, aiming for a better balance of Omega-3 and Omega-6 fats.

Autism and the immune system

Autism is a mysterious and heartbreaking ailment. Autistic babies don't respond to being cuddled and cared for. As toddlers and young children, they tend to live in a world of their own, seemingly indifferent to people but morbidly attached to objects. Comfortable only when endlessly repeating rituals, they usually appear overwhelmed by the noise and activity of normal childhood play. Many autistic children never develop speech; others use language oddly, repeating phrases over and over, or are unable to link thoughts through language.

In 1985, scientists at Stanford University discovered evidence placing autism in a category of ailments connected with an immune system abnormality. Researchers noted the presence of an unusual antibody circulating in the blood and spinal fluid of autistic children. This antibody attacks certain message receptors and interrupts normal nerve transmission in the brain.

Could the rise of autism be related to malnutrition? A 1978 double-blind study showed that autistic children improved when provided with vitamin B_6 and magnesium supplements, both pivotal nutrients for processing dietary EFA and converting them into prostaglandins. Could Omega-3 EFA in our diets be an important addition to brain functioning and the immune system? I think so.

How Omega-3 and diet affect teeth

Crooked, crowded teeth and an overbite (when the upper teeth come down too far over the lowers) are seen in the first teeth of tiny toddlers as well as older children. Suggested causes range from heredity to chronic thumb-sucking or mouth-breathing.

About fifty years ago, noted researcher and dentist Dr. Weston A. Price and his wife investigated the connection between diet and dental health in preindustrialized societies in which people were reputed to have few dental problems. Traveling to remote areas, they examined native people for signs of dental and other health problems. They took photographs and carefully recorded the food eaten in each region, wherever possible preserving samples for later nutrient analysis.

In *Nutrition and Physical Degeneration,* the Prices describe the men, women, and children they encountered as usually vigorous, healthy, and free of dental problems. To the Prices, the nutrition connection was unmistakable. Rampant tooth decay, along with diseases of modern society appeared wherever people abandoned traditional diets in favor of commercial foods sold at trading posts. The limited variety of foods sold were:

Hydrogenated (refined) vegetable fats	Refined sugar Refined flour	Canned goods Polished rice

The second generation on this food—the children of mothers who had abandoned the traditional diet for the store-bought foods—showed for the first time narrowed faces and jaws, pinched nostrils, overbite, and crooked, crowded teeth that were prone to decay.

Could the foods we eat affect our jaws and teeth in just a few short generations? Medical opinions vary, but we do know that fiber, vitamins, minerals, and polyunsaturated fats (Omega-3 and Omega-6) were more abundant in human diets 40,000 and even 100,000 years ago than today. Skulls of ancient people typically have generous facial bones with well-spaced teeth.

Contemporary anthropologists believe that the hunter-gatherers of thousands of years ago ate the same kind of diet that native people were consuming in preindustrialized societies at the time Dr. Price studied them. Evidence from fossil remains reveal wild game, fish, shellfish, berries, fruits, nuts, and vegetable foods such as roots, leaves, beans, and tubers comprising the basic diet, providing plentiful Omega-3 and Omega-6 EFA for our ancestors.

Native Foods
for a Healthy Pregnancy

Throughout their travels, Dr. and Mrs. Price were impressed by how primitive societies ensured ample nourishment for pregnant and lactating women. Here are some of the customs they recorded:

Eskimos of northern Canada. Salmon eggs were dried and eaten by women to increase fertility; salmon eggs were also an important food given to babies directly after weaning. Eskimos and Indians of Alaska ate fish, shellfish, marine plants, sea and land animals, and the organ meats of fish and animals. Plants and berries were eaten in season.

Indians of the Peruvian Andes. Natives often traveled hundreds of miles down the mountains to the sea coast to obtain supplies of fish eggs and kelp. (Sea products prevent the development of goiters, infertility, and other modernization diseases.) Peruvian Indians of the high Andes and plains ate the organs and meats of wild and domesticated animals, birds, fresh- and saltwater fish, and shellfish. They also gathered or grew a wide variety of plants, seeds, nuts, roots, and berries.

Amazon River Indians. These river and forest people ate freshwater fish, shellfish, small land animals, birds, wild plants, seeds, nuts, roots, and berries.

African tribes (cultures vary). Childbearing women ate carefully designated foods before pregnancy, as well as during gestation and lactation. In Kenya, Dr. Price reported, girls of the Kikuyu tribe "are placed on a special diet for six months prior to marriage. They nurse their children for three harvests." Inland agricultural African people sought freshwater fish and animals, meats and organs of animals, insects, and plant foods.

Fiji Islanders. Price reported that plant foods were carried from mountain areas at night and exchanged for sea foods provided by coastal natives. This was done by placing foods at appointed spots during the night, since the tribes were enemies. Despite their enmity, they knew tribal health depended on this secretive barter.

Melanesians, Polynesians, and Micronesians. These natives of the South Pacific enjoyed shellfish, sea mammals, marine plants, and land plants, including fruits, coconuts, seeds, and roots. Although coconut milk is very high in saturated fat, its consumption was balanced by rich sources of Omega-3 and Omega-6 polyunsaturated fats.

Australian aborigines. Natives of the Australian Outback ate large and small wild reptiles and other animals, insects, nuts, fruits, leaves, roots, and berries.

Gaelic people of the Outer Hebrides Islands of Scotland. Fish, shellfish, fish liver, oat cakes and porridge, barley, vegetables, and sea plants were part of a pregnant woman's diet.

Most of the societies studied by the Prices have changed beyond recognition in recent times because of industrialization. The evidence shows that when the diets of these people modernized, so did their diseases.

12
Omega Case Histories: Mental Illnesses Respond

The following are some case histories showing the effects of Omega-3 fatty acids on mental and physical well-being. Although the patients described here were clinically ill, their reaction to the Omega diets is relevant to everyone. If any of these case histories describe sensations you've felt, don't assume you are ill. But do visit your own physician, and discuss your symptoms as candidly as possible.

THREE SEVERE CASES OF SCHIZOPHRENIA

Restored calm and sleep

X., a twenty-six-year-old woman who had been a severe schizophrenic with hallucinations for ten years, also suffered from abdominal and gynecological problems, dry skin, tinnitus, dandruff, and many other problems. She had tried every medication, with little improvement. Mega-vitamin therapy and twice weekly dialysis had been beneficial but left her still very ill.

One-half hour after taking her first tablespoon of linseed oil supplement, she reported feeling calm. Within a few weeks, her hallucinations disappeared, her sleeping pattern became normal, and physical problems were much improved. X. had a narrow tolerance for linseed oil. Her ideal dosage was four tablespoons daily. If she took less, her illness worsened in a few days; more and she would develop "racing thoughts" indicative of a psychotic breakdown.

Family notes changes

Z., a twenty-eight-year-old male paranoid schizophrenic, suffered bizarre feelings of control. For example, he feared his watching television news reports would influence world events.

Z.'s optimal linseed oil dose was only one to two teaspoons daily. For the first time in years his paranoia diminished enough for his family to see remarkable changes. He was also sensitive to the exact dosage. If he took too much for a few days, he would also develop "racing thoughts." He was later helped by lithium.

Un-wired

L. was forty and had been schizophrenic for twenty years. She suffered from the delusion that she was controlled by invisible wires. L. weighed a hefty 200 pounds, and I put her on large doses of linseed oil: six to nine tablespoons a day. To this, as usual, I added a standard multivitamin antioxidant supplement.

After four months, her illness had not improved objectively, although her skin did. She was taken off the program. However, several months later L. approached me and begged, "Please, doctor, put me back on the oil. It takes the wires out of my head." It gave subjective relief from intrusive ideation.

RELIEF FROM AGORAPHOBIA

Phobics also get relief from anxiety through linseed oil supplements. The term *agoraphobia* comes from two Greek words: *phobos,* meaning fear, and *agora,* meaning marketplace or an open place of assembly. In this phobia, certain situations—usually being alone in open or unfamiliar places—trigger such unbearable anxiety and panic that phobics will structure their lives to avoid the anxiety-producing circumstances.

The following are less severe cases than those noted above, but the reactions to linseed oil supplements were just as dramatic, allowing these people to live fuller, happier lives.

Homebound man

K. was thirty-two years old and stayed home most of the time. For ten years, it was the only place in which he felt safe. His life was spent avoiding situations that might make him feel anxious. The psychiatrists who treated K. prescribed Valium daily.

One month after starting on a supplement of three tablespoons of linseed oil daily, K. reported feeling calmer and less anxious. After two and a half months he was sleeping better, and his attacks of anxiety were diminishing in length and frequency.

After a year, the anxiety had almost disappeared. On two occasions, while visiting relatives a considerable distance from home—in itself an achievement—K. went off the linseed oil for a week. He told me later he gradually began to feel tense, but after returning to daily oil supplements he once again became calm and less agitated.

Corner outing

A slender, thirty-five-year-old woman, M. had been housebound for eight years. Once or twice a month she would suffer severe anxiety attacks even without leaving her "safe places."

One month after starting on two tablespoons of linseed oil daily, her panic attacks ceased. Her anxiety lessened. At three months she told me she felt rested and calm and could leave her house, getting as far as the corner without panic.

Crossing the square

C. was another agoraphobic subject, fifty-eight years of age. An active attorney in government affairs, he had no problems leaving his home or traveling extensively when his job required it. But for forty years, whenever he crossed an open space—such as a city square—he panicked.

After three months of daily doses of three tablespoons of linseed oil, vitamin supplements, and a fiber-yogurt cocktail, C. felt less anxious and was able to walk across open spaces. At the same time, C. entered a behavior modification program to "retrain" his responses. He's now walking jauntily across open city areas, even though he still says it helps if he whistles.

Physical as well as mental relief

A great many of the mental cases I treated had physical problems— irritable bowel syndrome, joint diseases, tinnitus, food allergies—as well. I often saw improvement in both the mental and physical areas once the patient was placed on the Omega program.

MANIC-DEPRESSIVES
RESPOND TO OMEGA THERAPY

Sadness and depression are common human emotions. But in some people crippling despair becomes a way of life. It may be manic-depressive psychosis, which, like schizophrenia, seems to run in families. The mood disorder can take three different forms:

1. Cyclical unipolar depression, characterized by cycles of normal and deeply depressed moods. This is most common.

2. Bipolar manic-depressive disorder, characterized by cycles of depressed, normal, and highly elated, manic moods

3. Unipolar manic disorder, characterized by the mood swinging between manic and normal emotional states

The suffering of the depressed person in cyclical unipolar depression can be worse than any physical pain. Although the initial episode may be triggered by romantic disappointment, financial reverses, or death of a loved one, the despondency goes well beyond the limits of normal grief. This depression can also appear without any apparently stressful circumstances, leading many experts to think there is a physical component.

The bubbling elation of the manic phase in bipolar manic-depressive or unipolar manic disorder resembles the high of a drug addict. There is a nonstop flight of ideas and activity. The victim feels he or she is strong and powerful, but impatience and irritability can lead to an explosive psychotic state. Lithium is often useful in controlling the mood swings in bipolar and unipolar manic disorders, but relief is often incomplete.

Here are some case histories that describe what happened when manic-depressives took linseed oil supplements.

Modifying mood swings

Q., a twenty-nine-year-old woman who had been treated for bipolar manic-depressive psychosis for a year, did not respond well to lithium medication. She started on a supplement of one tablespoon of linseed oil daily, and within six weeks she felt much less tired. Her face looked fuller, her color seemed less pallid, and she felt less sensitive to cold.

However, she then had a severe depressive episode, with rapid mood swings from manic elation to agitation and depression. She abandoned the linseed oil supplement and her physical symptoms returned. It appears the right dose of linseed oil can help, while the incorrect dosage may cause mood swings. Dosages should be carefully monitored by a qualified professional whenever symptoms of any seriousness are apparent.

Self-help isn't always best

D., thirty-two years old, was incorrectly diagnosed for twelve years as suffering paranoid schizophrenia with severe depression. She took antipsychotic medication and medication for side-effects that developed from the primary medication: weight gain and hypothyroidism.

Placed on megavitamins—1 gram of niacin three times a day, plus B vitamins—by her psychiatrist, D. improved so remarkably that she was able to return to work for the first time in many years. However, her daily hallucinations and paranoia continued.

Because she weighed 220 pounds, I started D. on three tablespoons of linseed oil, in three divided doses, to be taken with her meals. After only four days she told me her fatigue had disappeared, and she felt elated. She raced through her housekeeping chores, and was once again able to enjoy gardening and other hobbies. She then increased her dose to a remarkable nine tablespoons daily, because it elevated her mood. While this erased her schizophrenia, she developed a typical manic attack—the first in her life—which disappeared on stopping the oil. This suggests she had an underlying manic-depressive disorder. By taking the proper linseed oil doses plus lithium, she now feels and behaves normally for the first time in ten years.

Feeling calm

H. was a forty-three-year-old homemaker and mother who had suffered from unipolar depression for six years. Lithium helped only a little, and she continued to suffer residual psychosis in the form of sudden violent thoughts.

While she remained on lithium, thyroid medication, and vitamins, I placed her on three tablespoons of linseed oil daily, and within one week she noticed that recurrent muscular pains had eased. By the seventh week, her violent thoughts disappeared and she felt calm—a feeling she had not enjoyed since the onset of the psychosis. She could no longer tolerate, nor did she need, her thyroid medication. However, excessive oil also induced a manic attack in this patient.

Omega-3 EFA—the common source of improvement

These cases are different in many ways, but a single thread runs through them all: Omega-3 fatty acids produced improved behavior, contributed to feelings of well-being, reduced psychotic thinking, and corrected many physical problems.

The beneficial response to Omega-3 indicates its importance to human mental health. As in traditional lore, fish, as well as northern plant foods, may indeed be brain food. We noted earlier that monkeys deprived of Omega-3 for a period of two years developed severe psychotic-like reactions and many other illnesses, and that rats performed poorly on maze tests, although only after a lifetime of deprivation. The results were echoed by those in the case of the young girl who developed severe neurological problems in just a few months when fed intravenously with low Omega-3 safflower as her only source of EFA. You'll recall that she recovered when given high Omega-3 soy oil. All this indicates that Omega-3 EFA, the most prominent EFA in the brain, is an essential nutrient of man—in fact, the one essential nutrient that distinguishes man and the primates from sub-primates.

B VITAMINS, PROSTAGLANDINS, AND YOUR MOODS

The human body needs vitamin B to process essential fatty acids and convert them to prostaglandins and other active lipids. A deficiency either of B vitamins or of essential fatty acids will affect the prostaglandins we make. The brain is not exempt from the effects of dietary deficiencies. Heredity probably determines our individual weak spots—how and where the unbalanced or deficient prostaglandins will affect brain circuits that control our thoughts, emotions, moods—and actions.

Today neuroscience can map the brain with some precision. Physicians can pinpoint which parts of the brain control movement, hearing, seeing, smelling and where emotions, mood, sexual drive, fear, rage, and anxiety are located, as well as what area of the brain produces pleasurable sensations. Clearly, nutritional deficiency will strike at the vulnerable centers, producing a large variety of different symptoms according to the point of susceptibility.

EFA help electrical nerve impulses

The long-chain Omega-3 acids are the most prominent unsaturated fats in the brain. These long-chain fatty acids provide the necessary fluid quality to the membranes of the nerve cells so that electrical nerve impulses can flow easily along the circuits of the brain. The prostaglandins made from the EFA are important regulators of nerve impulses.

When a dietary deficiency of Omega-3 EFA destabilizes the production of soothing prostaglandins, there tends to be a buildup of irritating inflammatory prostaglandins in the brain. They are similar to the prostaglandins that cause trouble in the bursae, joints, and digestive tract. In a susceptible person, the same process that causes spasms in the bowel may trigger spasms of irrational fears, panic, or rage when his or her brain is similarly affected. It may also trigger irrational feelings of euphoria.

We may view mental illness as an "irritable brain syndrome," a cousin of irritable bowel syndrome, irritable esophageal syndrome, irritable ear syndrome (tinnitus and Ménière's syndrome), and so on.

13

Omega Case Histories: Linseed Oil, Fish Oil, and the Heart

W hen linseed oil, fatty fish, or fish oils are introduced into the diet, they quickly bring promising changes in the blood and are responsible for better functioning of the cardiovascular system.

Hearts, strokes, and plaque

Each day people suffer heart attacks and strokes caused by atherosclerosis, a buildup of fatty substances in the arteries. The crisis trigger is the formation of blood clots that adhere to an injured artery wall; they are especially prone to attach themselves to places that are narrowed by plaques because of earlier problems. As the deposits accumulate, they block the flow of blood, and when major arteries of the body are involved—those serving the brain, heart, kidneys, and legs—a life-threatening problem results. A sudden spasm squeezing the arteries may also close down a partially blocked passage altogether.

Atherosclerosis often starts in the twenties, and the usual medical advice is:

- Stop smoking.
- Exercise.
- Reduce the fat in your diet.
- Lose weight.
- Avoid stress.

Other factors that burden the heart include:

- Chronically high blood pressure
- Poor collateral circulation
- Viscous blood that coagulates easily ("sluggish" blood)
- High sensitivity to cold
- Poor control of sodium excretion by the kidneys (chronic edema or swelling of tissues)

All of these factors are controlled by the EFA/prostaglandin regulatory system.

Slowing of accelerated blood clotting

Rapidly accumulating evidence indicates that certain fats—the Omega-3 fatty acids eicosapentaenoic acid (EPA), docosahexaenoic acid (DHA), and alpha linolenic acid (ALA)—are actually effective in lowering blood fats and reducing the tendency of blood platelets to stick together and pile up as clots on artery walls.

Positive test results with fish oils

Dr. William S. Harris and a group of researchers at Oregon Health Sciences report that a diet supplying EPA and DHA, both Omega-3 EFA, from salmon oil caused blood fats (triglycerides) to drop significantly lower than when Omega-6 oils—safflower and corn oil—were used in an otherwise similar diet. "Gram for gram, Omega-3 fish oil fatty acids were more effective in lowering cholesterol than were the Omega-6 fatty acids." Fewer calories of fish oil achieve the same or better effect than that of many southern plant oils; however, linseed oil has about the same benefits as fish oil.

While health improvements in the normal person on the salmon oil diet are impressive, changes in those suffering from inherited disorders that produce abnormally high fats and cholesterol in their blood (hyperlipidemia) were even more dramatic. The Portland researchers discovered that salmon oil produced these additional positive results:

• Prolonged—but still within the normal range—bleeding times
• Reduced number of platelets
• Decreased platelet adhesiveness

Similar results are obtained using supplements of linseed oil, which can:

• Normalize the blood pressure, reducing high blood pressure and elevating low blood pressure
• Normalize serum fats. (Niacin, fiber, and exercise also help to lower serum fats.)
• Reduce insulin requirements

We see here a synergistic system of effects.

My own view is that people with inherited disorders may fall into the broad classification of people who have a greater than average need for Omega-3 fatty acids. Their enzyme systems seem to favor processing the

Fish-Eating Eskimos
Suffer Few Heart Attacks

Greenland Eskimos are responsible for some of the excitement about fish oils. Danish and British scientists wondered how Eskimos could eat the highest fat diet in the world without getting heart attacks. So in 1976, researchers trekked to remote areas of Greenland to study Eskimos who still subsisted mainly on a traditional diet of fatty fish and blubber-packed seals.

Despite their huge fat intake, the Eskimos' blood was usually neither "sticky" nor viscous; cholesterol and fat levels in the blood were normal; and there was a low tendency for platelets to clump or collect in arteries. The standard "bleeding time" test showed that their blood took a very long time to clot. These discoveries explained their low rate of heart attacks and lack of blood clots in arteries.

Japanese living in Japan, unlike those living in the United States, also have a much lower incidence of heart disease and consume many times more fish and fiber. The fat in the fish and sea mammals that constitute a major portion of the Eskimo and Japanese diet is full of super-polyunsaturated Omega-3 (EPA and DHA). These fats provide the sea creatures, fish and mammals, with fluid membranes, flexible tissues, and temperature control—all advantages in Japan's and Greenland's icy waters.

The high Omega-3 content of the Eskimos' diets was reflected in a high content of the same fatty acids in the blood. It was many times higher than that of Europeans or Americans. Why? Was it racial? Was it genetic? Or did the high fatty acid levels in their blood depend entirely on diet? Could non-Eskimo people also profit from a diet high in Omega-3 EFA? Would these changes help or hurt the cardiovascular system?

The answers are encouraging: Studies show that Omega-3 fatty acids from fatty fish or fish oils are swiftly incorporated into the tissues regardless of race or age. The Japanese studies rule out racial and genetic factors and show that high Omega-3 EFA intake is the cause of low heart disease incidence in Japan. (And keep in mind that these people also have less arthritis, immune disease, schizophrenia, and all other modern maladies.)

The "Norwegian notch" phenomenon during World War II (see chapter 6) shows a similar pattern of response to a traditional diet featuring northern fish. There was also a 1968 study showing that linseed oil supplements, also high in Omega-3 EFA, significantly reduced the incidence of heart disease and related deaths. (See Appendix C for more details on this study.)

Omega-6 over the Omega-3 EFA. Consequently, they need large amounts of Omega-3 EFA to compete with the Omega-6 EFA. Genetic differences account for the different response (the disorder) to the same deficiency problem.

Thromboxane and prostacyclin—prostaglandins important in artery health

A prostaglandin known as thromboxane B_2 is needed to promote normal blood clotting; it prevents us from bleeding to death after a wound. Too much thromboxane B_2, however, constricts the arteries and forces blood platelets to clump together and adhere to artery walls, provoking thrombus and spasms leading to heart attacks or strokes. So the very factor that saves our lives by making blood sticky enough to stop flowing causes problems within the artery walls when the balance between Omega-6 and Omega-3 EFA is not correct.

Scientists have been searching for a way to help the human body avoid heart attacks and strokes—and at the same time not compromise the ability to stop bleeding. A 1984 study showed that a diet rich in either cod liver oil or mackerel (a very oily fish), which provides high Omega-3 EPA, caused thromboxane levels to fall, yet maintained full or higher than previous prostacyclin levels. Prostacyclin is a prostaglandin that inhibits platelet clumping in the blood. A more recent report has shown that as little as two fish meals a week—only a half pound to a pound of fish a week—can significantly reduce cardiac mortality.

Other benefits from fish foods

American researchers suggest that EPA and DHA may prove to be therapeutically useful in the prevention and treatment of atherosclerosis. German, Japanese, and British studies report similar findings. Both Japanese and British investigators found that adding Omega-3 EPA to the diet has the effect of reducing the viscosity of blood.

Viscous blood is often associated with diseased blood vessels in the feet, legs, and hands. Pain in the legs after walking a short distance (intermittent claudication) is a frequent sign of the problem. The researchers suggest that EPA reduces blood viscosity by changing red blood cell membranes, making them more flexible and allowing them to travel more freely through the narrowed blood vessels. My treatment with linseed oil supplements of two cases of long-term intermittent claudication, one of Raynaud's disease, and many involving general cold sensitivity have brought remarkable improvement.

Nutrition is a better answer than medication for heart patients

Nutritional treatment of heart patients shows that balanced Omega-3/ Omega-6 can be beneficial in avoiding or ameliorating heart problems. The practical effects are easy to see: Linseed oil, walnut oil, soybean oil, fish oils, and fatty fish or shellfish, cherished in traditional diets but excluded for the past twenty-five years from diets recommended for heart patients, are real life-savers.

The impact of the fish oil studies is all the more dramatic because of the simplicity of their findings. An inexpensive nutrient has succeeded where millions of dollars spent on drugs and biomedical research failed. But Omega-3 fatty acids positively affect more than the cardiovascular functions; they benefit the entire body as well.

Steps to fight heart disease

Abundant evidence shows that heart disease is particularly affected by the powerful synergistic effects of nutrition. Each of the following steps can reduce serum cholesterol. In combination, there will be an even more powerful effect promoting human health:

Supplements of EFA	Vitamin B_3 (niacin)
Dietary fiber	Exercise
Weight loss	Avoiding saturated fats

Since most diets are deficient in nutrients and overloaded with anti-nutrients, and since we tend to be overweight and exercise too little, correcting all these interacting factors at the same time is best. In fact, there is some evidence that lowering serum fats through diet and exercise can actually reverse atherosclerotic plaque formation. Think of it as a "cholesterol flush-away." I suspect that megadoses of Omega-3 oils in conjunction with the other health-contributing measures produce not only this cholesterol flush-away but also flush away isomer or funny fats and toxins (especially insecticides and other industrial chemicals that are lipid soluble and tend to accumulate in human tissues).

A REVIEW OF OTHER HEALTH RESPONSES TO THE OMEGA REGIMEN

We don't know the full extent of the illnesses that can be attributed to the modern disease of accelerated aging. The most common problems with which I have had some experience are

Immune disease	Bowel problems	Tinnitus
Heart ailments	Skin disorders	Neuralgias
Joint diseases	Mental illnesses	Obesity

Doubtlessly, many other disorders would fit into this group.

Physical responses

Several subjects in my study who had taken thyroid-stimulating medications for years, were able to stop medication; they no longer needed it. As PMS cases tend to show signs of hyperthyroidism, it would be reasonable to put PMS victims on the Omega program. Advice to this effect is also given by the American Heart Association, which recommends dietary therapy for hypertension in the hope of avoiding drugs that usually have unpleasant side-effects.

Insulin requirements have fallen dramatically in the two diabetics in the study.

A five-year menopausal anxiety-depressive syndrome that was inadequately treated with Premarin cleared up in a few months. And since there were no changes in blood estrogen levels, the effect was apparently not "estrogenic" but more likely "estroreceptogenic"—a normalization of prostaglandin estrogen receptor responses to estrogen. These findings suggest that extra vitamin D supplements together with the regular Omega program, might aid osteoporosis, which is related to estrogen deficiency.

Two individuals with Raynaud's disease who were part of the study responded well to the linseed oil regimen. This reaction was consistent with the reduced cold sensitivity in several cases in the study. All these benefits can be expected, given the cold-climate nature of the Omega-3 EFA.

In addition to skin conditions that have been helped, I've seen two cases of lifelong psoriasis, one mild and one severe, significantly ameliorated over a period of four to six months. Easy bruising that was unresponsive to all other nutritional therapy also responded.

A patient with incipient kidney stones and true renal colic, sporadically passing fine gritty material with blood clots for over a year, has now been symptom-free for several years on the Omega program.

A variety of neuralgias all cleared up in a month or so after years of trouble. There has been remarkable control of esophageal motor dysfunction; also relieved were irritable bowel syndrome, constipation, and hemorrhoids. Incipient pyorrhea as well as one case of early glaucoma seems to have been helped. Since tinnitus has been relieved, perhaps the related auditory problem of Ménière's disease will also respond, especially since it seems to be a modernization disease that is now increasing in incidence in Japan and elsewhere.

Mental responses

As well as improvement among subjects having classical psychoses and neuroses, as mentioned earlier, a chronic teen-age delinquent who was constantly in trouble at school and unresponsive to every other therapy—nutritional, medical, and psychological—reverted to normal behavior six weeks after linseed oil supplements were added to the rest of his nutritional supplement program.

In subjects who had developed symptoms of alcoholism, a sense of calm and a normal rather than addictive use of alcohol followed.

One of the schizophrenic cases who had seizures diagnosed as petit mal found that they disappeared along with major psychiatric problems after going on the Omega program.

Sexually transmitted diseases and sexual inclination

Since a wide variety of other immune disorders have been helped with the Omega regimen, it may also improve resistance to AIDS and herpes.

Some researchers believe that homosexuality may be related to abnormal hormonal influences on the developing fetus, so it would seem advisable for prospective parents to be especially careful about their diet. Significantly, the only person in the study who was homosexual also had a number of major health problems. The Omega program benefited all aspects of his health, although his homosexual preferences remained unaltered. To me, this indicates the deeply ingrained nature of that preference. However, borderline homosexuality may be influenced by the Omega program.

My findings seem to indicate that most illnesses that plague mankind today can be aided by correcting life-style and dietary factors, whether or not these factors are the primary cause of the particular illness.

The Comprehensive Mega-Omega Supplement Program

Part II presents the first comprehensive dietary supplement program that focuses on the role of EFA. This Mega-Omega regimen is designed to allow a person to find his or her own optimum supplement levels. Nutritional supplements, when taken for a period of some months, can ameliorate many overt illnesses.

For best results, this program should be used in conjunction with the Omega diets of Part III. These diets not only contribute essential nutrients but also remove many potent antinutrients present in the modern diet.

Since many factors affect health—food sensitivities, medicinal drug use, the level and type of dietary deficiencies, and individual genetic peculiarities—neither this supplement program nor anything else in this book can be viewed as a prescription for any individual. In any group, there is always someone with an unusual sensitivity. Therefore, you and your health professional must take responsibility for specific applications of the general principles given.

14
The Omega Supplemental Program for Overt Illness

B y this time I hope you can see how Omegafying your own diet may beneficially affect your general health. If you have any specific health problems, you might also be curious to see how much better Omegafying can make you feel. Here is a quick overview of the program—you'll see how simple and easy it is.

THE MINIMAL OMEGA SUPPLEMENTAL REGIMEN IN BRIEF

The following nutritional supplements will ensure a minimum of your requirements. It is especially important to consider supplements if you eat out often, use alcohol, consume considerable candy and soft drinks, or are suffering the general effects of aging or illness. Take this daily minimum, preferably in two or three divided doses with meals or in time-release form:

- A one-a-day 100 percent RDA multivitamin-multimineral supplement including selenium
- Calcium—1 to 2 grams of calcium carbonate or calcium gluconate. This is necessary because one-a-day supplements cannot accommodate the RDA of this macro-mineral. Take as one or two Tums or other supplement.
- A premeal mixed fiber-yogurt cocktail, which will provide a supplement of 10 to 20 grams of fiber daily (see page 106 for several fiber-yogurt cocktail recipes)
- Omega oils—one teaspoon food-grade linseed oil (about four capsules) or cod liver oil (about four capsules)

NOTE: You can experiment by increasing the oils, multivitamins and multiminerals every few weeks according to the plan below.

91

Consult your doctor before you go on any diet

For serious problems of any kind, consult your physician or nutritionist. Follow the basics given here to determine your version of the Standard Omega Program. Look at the table on pages 114–116, and note the nutrient deficiency that has been tentatively linked to your problem. Experiment with doses of specific nutrients you suspect are related to your illness. Many of my study subjects noticed improvement when they used a double dose of linseed oil every three days. But be cautious in moving to high dosages. Discuss them with your doctor or nutritionist to be sure of avoiding toxicity.

Avoid excessive mega-nutrients

Mega-nutrients can interact. I do not recommend taking limitless amounts of any nutritional supplement, because nutrients in mega-amounts can, like anything else, have adverse effects, and this is especially true when taking megadoses of several nutrients at once (see appended list of toxic side-effects on page 104). Be alert to any changes in your body functions. Megadoses interact with each other, so increase only one group of vitamin supplements at a time. If adverse effects appear, lower the dose or stop for a few days, then start again at a lower level.

Avoid "too much of a good thing"; don't overdose on any essential nutrient. Start with low—one RDA—doses. How do you know when you are taking too much? You can continue to increase your linseed oil or other essential nutrient intake gradually every three days. Stop if you notice any adverse effects, such as bloating, gas, dizziness, headache, or diarrhea. WARNING: In general a 150-pound person should not exceed

- One to two teaspoons cod liver oil *or* two to four tablespoons linseed oil (also available in capsules—ten capsules equal about one tablespoon) *or* one to five capsules of a fish oil such as Maxepa daily
- 25 milligrams of B vitamins
- 250 micrograms of selenium
- 600 IU of vitamin E
- One to 2 grams of vitamin C

Wait for improvement

Depending on your health circumstances, it may be several days to a week or several months before you see definable improvement. Once you recognize improvement, continue on your nutritional supplementation program for a year or more, but during this time, try gradually decreasing dosages as low as you can without incurring trouble again.

Continue your fiber supplement

Be alert to your digestive behavior. Adjust your mixed fiber-yogurt dose to between one teaspoon and one tablespoon at each routine meal to get odorless, well-formed coil bowel movements in twenty-four to forty-eight hours. If necessary, use Senekote or other vegetable-based laxatives for short periods. *Do not use laxatives regularly without checking with your physician.*

Exercise is important for any total program

Try to take an enjoyable level of aerobic exercise for thirty minutes at least three times a week, even if it's just vigorous walking (see Exercise Regimen, page 163).

Relax with friends and family

There is no way to measure stress—until you suffer the results. But you can avoid stress.

- Reduce stress with exercise or meditation (whatever works for you) or try situational counseling.
- Find an enjoyable job.
- Get one hug a day. (This is my minimum daily requirement. The RDA is two hugs, and three or more hugs a day is the therapeutic mega-dose.)

Stick to your diet—it will bring success

Continue on any existing medication that has been prescribed by your physician. Avoid over-the-counter medications. Should your health improve over weeks or months, you may find your need for medication and mega-nutrient supplements decreases dramatically. When this happens, continuing on the original prescription or continuing to take the same potent mega-vitamins can cause the appearance of toxic side-effects. As your need for medicine, drugs, or vitamin supplements decreases, you should reduce the amount you take proportionally. You are your own best guide, but also consult your physician.

A travel pack

There are supplement formulations well suited to the needs of people who travel a great deal. You can get fiber tablets—get those containing both cereal bran and fruit pectin or psyllium seed. You can also use fiber-yogurt granola-type bars. Capsules of linseed, fish, cod liver, Maxepa, and primrose oil are available in health foods stores, as are vitamin pro-A (carotene) and multivitamin-multimineral formulations with selenium. You can also easily take calcium tablets with you—e.g., Tums.

For the desperate

Patients whose illnesses do not respond satisfactorily to either the Omega Supplementation Program or the Standard Omega Diet, which removes antinutrients, should consider going on an Omega hypoallergenic diet (see chapter 21). They may be overwhelming their systems with unsuspected food allergens, which could be blocking all nutritional benefits.

THE SUPPLEMENTATION PROGRAM

The following mega-Omega supplement program was designed for anyone who suffers specific physical or emotional health problems, or who just wants to feel better. It can also improve the stamina of people whose zest for life outstrips their ability to keep going to the end of the day.

This supplementation program is designed to be combined with the regular Omega Diet given in Part III. It is the first supplementation program to be built around Omega-3 essential fatty acids—and thus the first *complete* supplement program. The goal is to normalize the ratio of Omega-3 to Omega-6 fatty acids in an average diet. The four phases of the program are:

Phase 1: Selecting and adjusting the linseed or other Omega-3 oil intake

Phase 2: Adding the cofactors of antioxidants, vitamins, minerals, and fiber

Phase 3: Maintaining the program.

Phase 4: Balancing the Omega-3 and Omega-6 EFA in the diet for optimum results

Phase 1: Selecting and Adjusting the Omega-3 Oil Intake

Find the best oil you can

The linseed oil suggested for use in all Omega diets is food-grade oil. Ideally it should be cold-pressed oil. But even if it isn't cold-pressed, it will still provide ample Omega-3 alpha linolenic acid and some Omega-6 linoleic acid. Examine the label and avoid a product that is partially or lightly hydrogenated. (**Caution:** *Don't confuse food-grade linseed oil with boiled linseed oil from paint and hardware stores.* Nutritional linseed oil is available in health food stores in most areas. If your store doesn't carry it, ask them to order it for you. It is listed in most health food catalogs. Be sure to get the oil in glass containers, not tin. Smell, then taste all oils before using them to be sure they are not rancid.)

Keep oil from becoming rancid

The linseed oil you buy should be in sealed, airtight bottles. The flavor should be nutty to slightly fishy—always fresh tasting. Refrigerate the oil as soon as the bottle is unsealed; it should keep well for several months in the refrigerator. Without refrigeration, it quickly becomes rancid after opening. Buy oil in pint quantities and use each bottle within a few months after opening.

Some people are concerned that linseed oil becomes rancid too rapidly to use. I offer my experiences, as well as those of the forty-four people in my pilot study and hundreds of colleagues, patients, and friends—and the evidence from laboratory tests. The danger of instant rancidity is highly exaggerated. This oil has passed the test of time. It has been used as a kitchen oil for thousands of years and was popular in dozens of countries with such varied climates as Russia and India. In addition, I have had the oil tested chemically and find no significant increase in oxidation products for two months after opening if kept under refrigeration.

What kind of oil is best?

Use only nonhydrogenated northern oils (no substitutes):

Linseed oil	Walnut oil
Soybean oil	Wheat germ oil
Chestnut oil	

Linseed oil is the best. The other oils are acceptable but not as high in Omega-3 EFA. Olive oil and sesame oil have little alpha linolenic acid but do have modest amounts of Omega-6. Although they have been used as food and cooking oils for centuries, use them only as a substitute for meat tallows and southern oils, not instead of the oils listed above. All southern oils—such as corn, cottonseed, olive, sesame, peanut, or safflower oil—are low in Omega-3 EFA.

Linseed oil and many of the other oils from plants indigenous to northern climates are also available in capsules or small perles*:

*Capsules of linseed oil, Maxepa (a fish oil), and Efamol (evening primrose oil) can be obtained via mail order from General Nutrition Corporation, 418 Wood Street, Pittsburgh, PA 15222. Tel: 800-457-2000.

• Ten large capsules equal about one tablespoon of linseed oil.
• Five small capsules, or perles, equal one large capsule.

Generally, one teaspoon of fish oil (four capsules) equals about one tablespoon of linseed oil, but their benefits can differ.

Finding the right dosage

The effectiveness of different oils can be different, so you must experiment, preferably starting with linseed oil. How nice it would be if I could tailor a program with just the right dosage of Omega-3 oils to suit everyone. That's impossible—each of us has a different need. However, here are guidelines for daily megadoses of linseed oil, developed from my pilot study.

Weight	Dosage
100 lbs.	Approximately 1 tablespoon
125 lbs.	Approximately 1–2 tablespoons
150 lbs.	Approximately 2–3 tablespoons
175 lbs.	Approximately 3 tablespoons
200 lbs.	Approximately 3–4 tablespoons

If there is any chance that you might be sensitive or allergic, start with one teaspoon (approximately four capsules) a day, and increase that dose gradually every four days. Remember, it may take a while to experience the desired benefits. Don't randomly increase dosages just because you aren't getting immediate results. When increasing dosages, stop if a side-effect develops that indicates you have reached your limit of tolerance. (NOTE: One tablespoon has approximately 100 calories, so you should cut calories elsewhere if you are concerned about weight gain.)

In my study, patients very often discovered a threshold dose was needed to achieve a therapeutic effect. For instance, there might be no tangible result from one teaspoon of linseed oil taken daily over many weeks or months. However, with an increase in dosage from one to two teaspoons, a complete remission of symptoms—of osteoarthritis, for example—might then be achieved in a few weeks. The smallest dose that worked for any subject was one-fourth teaspoon (one capsule) daily.

Oil toxicity

Before beginning, you should be aware of potential problems. Too much linseed or other oil over a long time can bring on the same symptoms as a deficiency of Omega-3. A few people may suffer diarrhea, sleepiness, muscle aches, or skin deterioration. It is a good idea to note any changes in your mood, skin, or stamina on a daily basis.

If your skin is dry, you should check it daily. When your dosage is adjusted correctly, your skin will develop a soft, slight sheen a few weeks after starting on the program—provided, of course, the rest of your nutrition is adequate. As a general rule, try to get 15 percent of your calories as protein, 55 percent as carbohydrates, and 30 percent as fat, with Omega-3 EFA as 1 to 2 percent of your total calories, Omega-6 EFA as 6 to 8 percent, and saturated fat at 10 percent or less.

Here are some additional guidelines:

- Two grams (one-half teaspoon of linseed oil) is the minimum daily requirement for any adult on a 2,000-calorie per day diet. If you take a smaller dosage, do not expect any therapeutic benefit.
- Four grams (one teaspoon) of linseed oil is the recommended daily allowance (RDA) for most adults in good health who are not suffering any overt Omega-3 deficiency symptoms. Since there are about 10 calories per gram in linseed oil, this will contribute only about 2 percent of the recommended calorie intake for a 150-pound person who is not doing strenuous work (2,000 calories).
- Those who suffer ailments related to Omega-3 deficiency may find they need much more than four grams of linseed oil for a period of months.
- One to four tablespoons was needed daily for the first few months by most of the subjects in my pilot study. This translates into about three to twelve teaspoons, or ten to forty capsules. Only by constantly monitoring, adjusting, and experimenting could we determine each subject's optimal dose. You must be prepared to develop your own program. Increase your dosage gradually every few days and try to take oils and all other supplements in divided doses with meals or in time-release form.
- Be alert to any changes in all body reactions—either good or bad effects. If you note these changes, respond to them. Good results mean you should continue the dosage at the present level. Bad results require stopping for several days and then beginning again at a lower level.

When and how to take the oil supplements

Linseed oil should be taken with meals whenever possible, preferably in divided doses. Some subjects take it neat, others prefer to follow the oil with orange juice. Capsules or perles of linseed oil may be more convenient. To make the large capsules easy to swallow, soften them in warm water for a few minutes before attempting to swallow them.

You can also stir linseed oil into soup or other liquid food; it can be used in vinaigrette dressings (see recipes in Part III). Use whatever method lends itself to taking measured amounts with ease and con-

When to Expect Benefits from Omega-3 Supplements

The following were typical periods of time in which subjects of the pilot study noted the beneficial effects of the Omega-3 linseed oil supplements. A long wait is not always necessary before results are visible:

Time after taking oil supplement	Reaction
2 hours	Mood improved, feeling of calm, depression relieved
2–7 days	Skin smoother, with less flaking and scaling; backs of hands and fingers smoother
2–14 days	Fewer hallucinations; relief for disturbed mental patients; relief from feelings of anxiety.
2–6 weeks	Osteoarthritis relieved, with easier movements and less inflammation and pain Bursitis and other soft-tissue inflammations reduced Tinnitus and noises in the ears subside Dandruff and flaking of the scalp less noticeable; dry skin alleviated
2–4 months	Rheumatoid pain diminished "Easy bruising" reduced Choking spasms subside Fewer muscular spasms; no nighttime leg cramps; relief from ocular spasms Relief from itching and burning sensations Improved skin color Reduced sun sensitivity
3–6 months	Diminished food allergies Healing of chronic infections Disappearance of rough, bumpy skin on upper arms Improved alcohol tolerance Improved cold tolerance Lessening of fatigue Increased calm and feeling of well-being

As you can see from this table, the response time can vary from hours to days, weeks, or months. Improvement in some cases can continue for up to one or two years before leveling off. Allergies often require a long time for improvement. Nothing is guaranteed, because each person's makeup is so individual. Persistent emotional or physical problems may improve only after several months—if at all.

venience. It is important to make taking the supplement dosage a regular practice.

If you suffer gallbladder or digestive problems related to fat metabolism, taking two or three soy lecithin capsules along with the linseed oil may help. The lecithin can help emulsify the linseed (or other Omega) oil, allowing it to be absorbed with less discomfort. As a bonus, soy lecithin has the Omega-3/Omega-6 content of soy oil.

Phase 2: Adding the Cofactors—Antioxidants, Vitamins, Minerals, and Fiber

The Omega-3 nutrients are not the only nutrients missing from the average American diet. Vitamins, minerals, and fiber are also missing. To achieve the optimum results from your Omega diets, it is necessary to add these cofactors either at the beginning or after a few weeks. Vitamins, minerals, and fiber work to amplify the effects of Omega oil and vice versa. The benefits are often not added, but multiplied synergistically—the total is more than equal to the sum of the factors.

What are cofactors?

As the Omega-3 EFA become part of your tissues, they need to be protected by antioxidants—vitamins, minerals, and other dietary supplements that retard oxidation. (Oxygen can affect the way your tissues respond and age, very much as it acts to form rust on iron.) Here is how many of the essential nutrients work together:

- Antioxidants—in particular, vitamins pro-A, A, C, and E and selenium and cysteine—protect the EFA from oxidation.
- Fatty acids need enzymes to transform them into forms suitable for body use, notably the regulatory EFA such as the prostaglandins.
- Enzymes need B vitamins and minerals before they can work on fatty acids.
- Fiber is a cofactor because it controls fat and cholesterol metabolism in the bowel, which in turn changes blood cholesterol and the need for EFA.

To make the Omega program work, any existing nutrient deficiency must be resolved at the same time that you fill your Omega-3 reservoirs. You must overcome all deficiencies—bring yourself to a normalized level—before you can see the greatest therapeutic benefit, and you must reduce antinutrients.

For fast results

For the fastest results, undertake together Phase 1—selecting and adjusting the linseed oil intake—and Phase 2, adding the cofactors of vitamins, minerals, and fiber. In any case, you should start Phase 2 within three or four weeks after starting Phase 1—or at any time after you introduce linseed oil into your diet. Some people prefer to delay the start of vitamins, minerals, and fiber, so they can track and note their progress on the oil supplement alone. But for best results both are needed: oil supplements and cofactors.

How the Omega-3 Supplement Program affects other nutrients

On the Standard Omega-3 Diet or linseed oil program, many people who receive the benefits at low vitamin doses of only about one RDA or slightly higher may suffer mildly toxic problems with high doses because of the synergy between the nutrients. The toxicity effects are generally reversible. When in doubt, stop taking the supplements for a few days and start at lower doses. Also consult your physician or nutritionist.

VITAMIN COFACTORS

THE B VITAMINS: PROCESSORS OF EFA

What and why. As Omega-3 EFA enter your tissues, you may find that modest supplements of the B vitamins can aid you. Retest as the months go by to find the lowest doses that give you the optimum results. If you now take B vitamins, either in a daily multivitamin or in a B-complex supplement, you may find you must reduce your present supplements as your deficiency of Omega-3 oil is overcome. The beneficial effects you previously felt from vitamin B supplements may come about, in part, because they boosted the action of the Omega-3 EFA in your body.

How much. If you've never taken vitamin supplements, begin with the major B vitamins—B_1 (thiamine), B_2 (riboflavin), B_3 (niacin), B_5 (pantothenic acid), B_6 (pyridoxine), B_{12} (cyanocobalamin), folacin, and biotin—in amounts from approximately one to ten times the RDA (Recommended Daily Allowance). Start at the lower level and gradually work up. Here are the recommended amounts:

Megadosing with B Vitamins

Vitamin	RDA	Recommended for initial megadosing
B$_1$ (thiamine)	2 mg.	5–6 mg.
B$_2$ (riboflavin)	2 mg.	5–7 mg.
B$_3$ (niacin)	20 mg.	100 mg.
B$_5$ (pantothenic acid)	10 mg.	50 mg.
B$_6$ (pyridoxine)	2 mg.	6–8 mg.
Folacin (folic acid)	0.5 mg.	1 mg.
Biotin	0.1 mg.	0.5 mg.
B$_{12}$ (cyanocobalamin)	5 mcg.	50 mcg.

NOTE: The RDA is a minimal level for those in poor health, and the major B vitamins have been used in high doses for long periods of time with a good safety record. While excessive amounts, especially of vitamin B$_6$, can cause trouble, that is unusual, and stopping reverses the trouble in nearly all cases. Most normal people will get a niacin flush with 50 to 200 mg. of niacin—a flushing and tingling of the face and ears for a few minutes.

The actions of vitamin B$_6$ (pyridoxine) appear to play a pivotal role in the making of prostaglandins. Supplements in amounts considerably over the RDA have had beneficial effects on diseases similar to Omega-3 deficiency diseases: arthritis, premenstrual tension, and heart disease. Foods that are good sources of the B vitamin are yeast, wheat germ, liver, fish, legumes, milk, and eggs.

VITAMIN A

What and why. Vitamin A comes from both plant sources and fish liver. Beta-carotene, which is also known as pro-vitamin A, comes only from plants. It is an antioxidant working with vitamins C and E and selenium to protect the EFA. The health of skin and mucous membranes throughout the body depends on a diet that is adequate in vitamin A and pro-A. They are also essential for normal vision and healthy teeth, gums, and sex glands. A lack of A will show up in dry, scaly skin and visual problems. Cancers of the gastrointestinal tract and lungs have been produced in animals deficient in this vitamin.

How much. There is no evidence of problems involved in the consumption of food containing large amounts of carotene, from which the body makes its own vitamin A. However, you can get too much vitamin A from fish liver oils, so keep cod liver intake down to one to two teaspoons daily.

Some people who eat large amounts of carotene-containing foods (oranges, carrots, dark leafy vegetables, and deep colored fruits) have noticed that their skin seems to turn yellowish. I recommend taking 10,000 IU of pro-A and never more than 20,000 units, especially when on high oil doses.

In supplement form, be very wary of this vitamin—50,000 units a day can result in the symptoms of toxicity in a few months. These symptoms include headaches, fainting, nausea, joint pains, diarrhea, and skin problems.

VITAMIN C

What and why. Vitamin C is a potent antioxidant that protects tissues from damage. Controversy still rages over the amount to take as supplements. The RDA is set at about 50 milligrams for adults, but some scientists feel that high intake can be useful in combatting cancer, the common cold, hepatitis, and other viral disorders. There are also studies indicating it can lower blood cholesterol.

How much. For people without kidney problems, I see no danger in starting at 500 milligrams of vitamin C and gradually increasing the daily dosage to 1,000 milligrams. Foods rich in vitamin C include many fruits, especially citrus. In rare cases, large doses (overdoses) can contribute to the development of kidney and bladder stones.

VITAMIN E

What and why. Vitamin E is also an antioxidant. It keeps oils from going rancid and does a similar job of protecting the EFA in our tissues from oxidative damage. Taking the additional oil on the Omega Diet means that more unsaturated fatty acids are being deposited in cell membranes. As a sensible precaution, supplements of vitamin E should be taken along with other antioxidants—vitamins pro-A, A, C, and selenium, because they interact. Foods rich in vitamin E include wheat germ, wheat, avocado, green leafy vegetables, and sweet potatoes. Seeds and nuts that contain unsaturated oils often are good sources of vitamin E (as well as of other nutrients).

How much. I recommend taking 50 to 100 IU of vitamin E—never more than 600 units. There are reports of clotting problems and phlebitis if high levels are taken. There is, in fact, a pro-oxidant effect produced by excess antioxidants.

THE MINERAL COFACTORS

The toxic levels of most trace elements are very close to the required level. Some of these minerals are very potent, even in very small amounts. In addition, large doses of one mineral may suppress absorption of other nutrients. For example, a very high copper intake (more than 20 milligrams per day) has been found to interfere with zinc absorption.

CALCIUM

What and why. This is the most abundant mineral in the body and it is responsible for many vital functions. The importance of maintaining the strength of bones and teeth is obvious: Low calcium is linked with osteoporosis. Also, when in proper balance with other minerals—sodium, potassium, and magnesium—calcium helps regulate the rhythmic contractions and relaxation of heart and other muscles.

How much. It is generally recognized that only about 30 percent of the calcium you eat daily is actually absorbed. Large amounts of fiber in the diet, the use of laxatives, consumption of large amounts of protein, or drinking several cups of coffee daily can all interfere with the absorption of calcium.

A minimum for women is about 1,200 milligrams a day. Because this amount of calcium cannot be fitted into a one-a-day multivitamin/multimineral supplement pill, you must take calcium supplements separately. Taking two Tums tablets a day is one way to get your requirement. Too high an intake of calcium—several RDAs—can cause kidney stones.

SELENIUM

What and why. The trace mineral selenium, when taken with vitamin E, appears to have a special role as an antioxidant in guarding the EFA in cell membranes. Veterinarians now believe deficiencies of selenium in livestock in the United States and Canada are common. This may result from depletion of the soil in certain parts of the country.

While plants need many of the same minerals that animals and people do, plants don't usually require selenium, so crops can grow well in lowselenium soil. However, those crops will be selenium-deficient from our viewpoint. Further along the food chain, people and livestock who eat the plants grown in this soil do not get the needed selenium in their foods. These low-selenium areas are mainly in the far west and east.

How much. A high intake of polyunsaturated fats raises the selenium requirements. The RDA is set tentatively at 50 to 200 micrograms; I recommend a supplement of from 5 to 25 micrograms if taken in the chelate form. Determine your own tolerance level.

OTHER ESSENTIAL TRACE MINERALS

What and why. In addition to vitamins pro-A, A, E, and C and selenium, the minerals copper, zinc, and manganese are also antioxidants.

The amino acids methionine and cysteine are also mineral antioxidants. They are found in protein foods.

How much. Because these minerals are needed only in small (trace) amounts, a complete one-a-day type of multivitamin and multimineral supplement provides sufficient amounts as a start for most people.

Potential Toxic Effects of Nutrient Supplements

When you take nutrition supplements you should be very aware that vitamins and minerals are powerful. They can help, but they also can produce undesired toxic effects. The most usual negative result of megadoses is to reinduce the original illness for which you took the nutrients. Specific toxic effects are:

- Vitamin A, 25,000–50,000 IU—headaches, fainting, dry skin, hair loss, fatigue. Women at risk for pregnancy should not take more than 8,000 IU daily.
- Niacin, 100 mg. or more—immediate skin flush
- Vitamin C, 1–2 grams (over many months)—burning on urination, skin rashes, kidney stones
- Vitamin D, 25,000 IU—dizziness, diarrhea, nausea, fatigue, kidney stones
- Vitamin E, over 600 IU—increased blood pressure, clotting
- EFA, over 1–3 teaspoons (long term); B vitamins, 10–100 RDA—sleepiness; headache; skin roughening on fingers, knuckles, heels; muscle aches
- Copper, 40 mg.; iron, 100 mg.; magnesium, 2.0 grams—various symptoms
- Iron, chronic overload—arthritis, impotence
- Magnesium, over 1 gram—diarrhea
- Selenium, 500 mcg.—garlic breath, eczema, neurological problems

---

Adverse nutrient interaction effects

Because the essential nutrient interaction is synergistic, when nutrients are taken in excessive amounts, not only can they produce the toxicity effects indicated in the box, they may also produce relative deficiencies of the other essential nutrients. Certain of these nutrient-induced nutrient deficiencies are documented:

- Too much fiber or unleavened cereals or beans can induce mineral deficiencies of calcium, zinc, or iron because these foods contain phytic acid, a chelator. However, phytic acid is destroyed by cooking and leavening, and this adverse effect has never been reported in people on a reasonably balanced diet.

- Too much flaxseed can produce a vitamin B_6 deficiency, acrodynia, because it contains a B_6 inhibitor. However, this effect is unknown in those who consume a balanced diet and take only a few teaspoons of flaxseed daily, as in Roman bread or spread over cereals or meat, a tradition in some families going back to ancient times.
- Too much of any of the divalent minerals—calcium, zinc, or iron—can depress the absorption of the others. This is another reason why megadosing with one nutrient should not be continued for long periods of time without balancing the others.
- Too much vitamin B can induce a relative deficiency of EFA, provided the EFA intake is marginal. Conversely, too much EFA can induce a relative B-vitamin deficiency if the diet is marginal in B vitamins.
- Too much EFA can induce a relative deficiency of EFA antioxidants—vitamins pro-A, C, and E and selenium.
- Too much of one antioxidant can induce a relative deficiency of the others, because they also work synergistically. This is why large doses of vitamin C should be covered by supplements of the other antioxidants if continued for long periods of time.
- Too much of any of one of the fifty or so essential nutrients can induce not only its own toxicity effect but can also induce a relative deficiency of the remainder.

All of these effects are rare in those who are eating sensibly; when they do occur, they are usually reversible and are mild in comparison to the extremely dangerous side-effects and toxicities produced by medicinal drugs.

THE FIBER COFACTOR

Look back at chapter 4. Fiber is important in all diets—it is especially important when you are in Phase 2 of the Omega Supplemental Program. The foods that sustained our ancestors were high in fiber. Most of the fiber comes from:

Raw fruits and vegetables	Beans	Oatmeal
Kasha (buckwheat)	Millet	Potatoes
Whole-wheat cereals	Yams	Coarse breads
Thick vegetable soups		

Today's processed food is scant in both Omega-3 EFA and fiber. Deficiencies in both these important features of our modern diet compound all nutritional problems. Although fiber is not yet officially considered an essential nutrient, even the orthodox are hinting at a connection between serious ailments and fiber deficiency. The Omega Diet includes a yogurt-fiber premeal appetizer or "cocktail" with every meal (see page 29 for the recipe). The serum cholesterol–lowering effects of the hydrophilic fibers psyllium and pectin work with the cereal bran to improve bowel movements.

How fiber normalizes the digestive tract

Within two or three days after you start taking the fiber-yogurt appetizer, it should produce an "odorless coil" bowel movement. If you get a poorly formed stool, reduce the amount of fiber at each meal by about ¼ tablespoon.

You might feel bloated or gassy for about a week as changeovers take place in the bacteria of your digestive tract. The yogurt provides your digestive system with aerobic bacteria—the "good guys"—that will improve the health of the colon. These bacteria thrive on high-fiber foods, driving out odor-producing anaerobic bacteria—the "bad guys."

Mixed Fiber in Bulk
(28 servings)

2 cups (4 ounces) miller's bran
¼ cup (1 ounce) psyllium seed powder
1 tablespoon (¼ ounce) pectin powder (optional)

Mix well. Store dry, sealed, in cool place.
To serve: Add 1 rounded tablespoon mixed fiber to yogurt and water as per single serving directions. (You can also add ¼ teaspoon wheat germ to each single serving if you wish.)

Other Fiber Formulas

• 1 tablespoon bran plus 1 teaspoon pectin or 1 teaspoon psyllium powder
• 1 tablespoon bran plus 1 teaspoon each of pectin and psyllium
• 1 tablespoon bran plus one capsule of glucomannan

Combine any of the above formulas with plain yogurt before taking. If you have problems with spasms in your esophagus, avoid glucomannan because it can swell and block the esophagus. If this happens, swallow small amounts of warm water to encourage the glucomannan to dissolve and move—either up or down.

Substitutions because of allergies.

If you are allergic to milk, substitute low-sugar applesauce in place of yogurt. Take the premeal fiber mixed in water or fruit juice instead of yogurt, or take acidophilus capsules instead. You may also make these substitutions:

- Use honey sparingly, or use fructose or sugar substitutes if necessary.
- If you have colitis, start with small amounts and work up to the suggested amount. Drink a glass of water with each fiber supplement. Also cook all vegetables and fruit thoroughly.

Phase 3: Maintaining the Program

After Phase 1, introducing Omega oil into your diet, and Phase 2, adding the cofactors to increase the benefits of the Omega supplements, the next step is to monitor yourself and evaluate your response to the "Omegafied" supplement program. This step is more important than with any other nutrition program, because Omega-3 EFA are metabolized differently by every person—and because you are now on the first nutritionally complete supplement program. You will be receiving the full synergistic benefits and, for this reason, are susceptible to enhanced toxicity effects.

The goal is always to take the minimum amount of supplements that works and then to phase them out—or down—after a time, letting the Omega Diet carry you. After all, on this diet you will be getting five to ten times the Omega-3 and other nutrients in your previous diet.

Looking through the skin window

The skin provides a window on our internal well-being. I find skin response a convenient guide for discovering what levels of Omega-3 linseed oil and what cofactors work best for most patients. Working together, we often adjust the linseed oil dose to try to get a visible reduction of skin dryness in three to four weeks. The resultant smoothing of the skin, added sheen to the hair, and brightening of the eyes are delightful to see and are sure evidence that something good is happening throughout the body.

How skin texture can serve as a nutrition guide

Many people with very dry skin on their hands, feet, and body ironically have excessive oil on their forehead, eyebrows, scalp, and nose. The oil from overactive sebaceous glands causes greasy scales and dandruff. This problem is called seborrheic dermatitis and is related to an Omega-3 deficiency. Seborrheic dermatitis tends to normalize on the Standard Omega-3 Program. As the hands and feet become smoother and softer, the skin of the scalp is freed from scales. Once my patient subjects find the linseed oil and cofactor doses that produce the best results for them, they stay on their own personal programs for at least two or three months, or until their skin shows substantial improvement.

Adjusting your dosage

In my experimental group, when we were unable to achieve a positive change I suspected:

- Too little linseed oil—the dose was increased
- Cofactor deficiency—vitamin supplements were increased
- Cofactor excess, such as too high an intake of B vitamins or vitamin A—the vitamin dosage was reduced

You should consider possible reasons for no response. Could it be that the enzymes that transform alpha linolenic to EPA and DHA are not working efficiently? In that case, substitute fish oils—such as cod liver oil, Promega, or Maxepa—which contain EPA and DHA fatty acid, for the linseed oil.

Still another possible reason for a lack of response could be poor absorption of the oils and cofactors. If you suspect this, your physician or nutritionist may be able to help you solve this problem. A series of tests done by a professional will reveal absorption problems. If you have such problems, you should correct them and possibly carefully increase the difficult-to-absorb vitamin and mineral cofactors.

Maintaining the program with the lowest possible dosage

Oil. After three months on the regimen, while keeping the cofactors steady and other fats and oils in the diet as low as practical, I asked the patients in my experimental group to reduce linseed oil by half for a few weeks. If previous problems did not recur and no new problems manifested themselves, the patients were asked to reduce the dose by half again. This dosage lowering continued until the original symptoms reappeared. In this way patients could stabilize at the lowest effective dose of linseed oil. Another way to lower Omega-3 is to switch to supplements of walnut or soy oil, which have a lower Omega-3 EFA content.

Vitamin and mineral cofactors. After a few weeks, while holding the linseed oil level steady, my patients reduced cofactor vitamin and mineral doses in half for a few days, or a week, and carefully noted the response. Again, this is the way to find the lowest effective dosage.

Every few months my patients used this same technique to recheck both the oil and cofactor doses. As long-term healing took place, the requirements for oil, vitamins, and minerals often declined. It is important to explore to find the lowest effective dose for each person as time goes by. The original dose can be too strong for a long-term program—a dosage level that helped originally actually causes a toxic reaction later on. (NOTE: Your medication may do the same thing.) A very few subjects in the pilot study still required three tablespoons of linseed oil daily after two years on the diet. But for most the requirements dropped drastically. Usually, the drop in required dosage was evident from one to six months after starting the program; the benefits of the Omega program also were greatest by then.

Phase 4: Balancing the Omega-3 and Omega-6 Groups

The final phase of the Standard Omega-3 Program completes the formula:

(Omega-3:Omega-6) + vitamin and mineral cofactors + fiber = Good Health

This "fine-tuning" requires that you gradually explore the optimum ratio of different oils.

Balancing with the Omega-6 oils

Start by substituting about half the linseed oil you have been taking with safflower oil. Continue to increase the safflower oil and decrease the linseed oil until you see a change in your skin or general health.

Another way is to switch to walnut or soy oil, which have a lower ratio of Omega-3 to Omega-6. You must be alert for any change, either for the better or for the worse. Keep asking yourself, Is my skin getting softer and smoother? Do I feel better or not? As Dr. Richard Kunin, author of *Mega-Nutrition: The New Prescription for Maximum Health, Energy, and Longevity* and *Mega-Nutrition for Women,* says, "Listen to your body."

This continued experimentation and evaluation will guide you in working out an optimum ratio of Omega-3/Omega-6 oils—and the minimum supplement amount—that is best for you. Recheck every few months to keep your balance perfect.

Climate changes and the Omega-3 oils

Because of their super-polyunsaturated nature, higher amounts of Omega-3 oils are required in cold climates than in warm climates (and more are produced by the cold-climate food chain). Thus, there is a north-south balance between supply and demand—if not distorted by hydrogenation or transportation. The Omega-3 EFA provide cell membranes and tissues with extra flexibility, something that is otherwise reduced in cold weather.

Balancing with fish oils

If after a few months on linseed oil you feel the need for further improvement, you may want to explore benefits from fish oils, as these directly deliver the super-polyunsaturated EPA and DHA to your body. While alpha linolenic acid in linseed oil can be transformed into EPA and DHA by your body's enzymes, if either your body doesn't create the right enzymes or the enzymes do not do an efficient job, you may get the benefit you want by adding cod liver or another fish oil to your diet. EPA can turn into prostaglandins that are beneficial to the cardiovascular system and other cell membranes. DHA is the most polyunsaturated fat and is vital for healthy brain, eyes, and sex organs. Fish oils have almost no Omega-6 gamma linolenic and very little Omega-3 alpha linolenic.

To explore the use of fish oils, gradually work up to the following amounts of fish oil in your diet in place of linseed oil:

- One teaspoon (four capsules) of cod liver oil, *or*
- Up to six capsules daily of Maxepa or Promega, a fish oil concentrate of EPA and DHA

Begin by reducing the linseed oil in half while substituting with one-third to one-half of the maximum dose of fish oil. Adjust gradually every week or so until you find the optimum amount. *Do not exceed one teaspoon of cod liver oil* (because of its high vitamin A content).

A combination of fish and vegetable oils may be most effective in slowing down the production of "bad" prostaglandins—those responsible for menstrual cramps and for feelings of emotional turmoil—and encouraging the "good" prostaglandins that enable cells to heal and provide a feeling of calm and well-being.

Evening primrose oil

Another way to balance the Omega-3 and Omega-6 oils is to take evening primrose oil, which is high in gamma linolenic acid (GLA). GLA can sometimes mimic the effects of Omega-3 oils through complex metabolic interactions. Evening primrose oil can be bought in health food or drugstores. (A reliable brand is Efamol.)

Start with a few capsules a day and work up to four or six capsules daily. British researcher Dr. David Horrobin and other scientists have recorded the therapeutic benefits of this Omega-6 oil. Like Omega-3 oils,

evening primrose oil can direct the activity of the "good" prostaglandins.

Several of my pilot study patients found that taking evening primrose oil alone aggravated their health problem but that it was helpful when combined with linseed oil and/or fish oil. Only testing will tell what balance works best for you.

Sufficient vitamin and mineral cofactors can make a difference

If a primate is deficient in the antioxidant element selenium, providing supplemental essential fatty acids will only make the selenium deficiency worse. Whatever selenium stores are in the body will be used up that much sooner in an attempt to protect the EFA from oxidative damage.

In the same way, linseed and/or fish oils on the Standard Omega-3 Program may make health symptoms worse over a period of weeks and months—unless sufficient vitamin, mineral, and fiber cofactors are available on a regular basis. Conversely, overdosing on B vitamins or other cofactors can wipe out your EFA supplies unless you supplement properly with them.

Too much oil can cause a return of health problems

I've mentioned this already, but it bears repeating: After some months of steady improvement on the balanced Standard Omega Program, an excess of Omega-3 oil or any other supplement may reintroduce your original problems. Researchers find that laboratory animals will show clear deficiency symptoms in their fur and skin from too little EFA, but when they give the animals ten times the indicated amount of EFA, the same symptoms show up.

I have learned through experience that if I see a toxic effect, such as dry skin, confusion, loss of hearing—or whatever seems to be the problem—it generally means that the person has simply turned the dial up too hard. Modifying the oil dosage or increasing the selenium or vitamin E supplements upward *(if they were low)* gradually restores the previous gains and brings the patient back to comfortable health.

Flare-up of cysts

Secretions of skin and other organs are often normalized on the Omega-3 Supplemental Regimen. Pre-existing cystic conditions such as endometriosis may clear up, or plugged ducts of the skin, ovaries, or elsewhere may spontaneously open, making surgical relief unnecessary. However, the reverse sometimes occurs if the cyst outlets remain completely blocked and secretions increase. In that case, only you can judge if the benefits warrant continuing with the program. Stopping the oil usually provides relief.

SAFETY MARGIN
FOR LINSEED OIL THERAPY

The safety margin for linseed oil EFA therapy is high compared with most medications and drugs. It takes about ten times the therapeutic dose before toxic symptoms appear. This safety margin is similar to that for vitamin A. A deficiency of vitamin A causes skin pathology, dry mucous membranes, and weak gums, and the same symptoms appear in toxic overdoses when the amount taken is ten times or more the normal dose.

Some Identified Toxicity Effects of Mega-EFA and Other Mega-Nutrients

Taken over many months, too much of any of the oils or other essential nutrients can reintroduce the original symptoms or produce the following easily reversible effects:

- Sleepiness, tinnitus, mild headache, palpitations, lymph node tenderness
- Hand eczema, knuckle and heel roughness, fingertip peeling, acne, and either excessive oiliness or dryness of the hair
- Enlargement of existing skin and possibly ovarian cysts with blocked ducts
- In patients with overt psychosis, excessively high doses may induce racing thoughts in schizophrenia and hypomania in manic-depressives, including unipolar depressives.
- Mild diarrhea
- Myopathy, bursitis, tendonitis, arthritis
- Any of the toxic side-effects of concurrent medication

NOTE: In rare cases, an individual may be sensitive to essential nutrients or impurities in them. Some people are sensitive to selenium at 10-microgram levels when taken in purified form. A sensitivity to flaxseed or fish oils is rare, but you should be aware of such possible allergic reactions as flushing, dizziness, edema of the throat (tightening or choking sensation), or eczema.

Many of these effects result from an imbalance in the ratio of essential nutrients and can be relieved either by stopping the supplements for a few days and restarting at lower levels or by increasing the appropriate conutrients to bring their synergistic effects into optimal balance. For example, if too much oil is suspected, either reduce the oil intake or increase one or more of the antioxidants or the B vitamins to help your body process the oil. If you are taking any medication, you may be seeing their side-effects and need to reduce medication doses rather than nutrients. Check with your physician.

Linseed oil and medications

Linseed oil, ibuprofen, aspirin, and steroids such as cortisone all have an effect on prostaglandin production. But each has a side-effect:

- Excessive aspirin can cause tinnitus and stomach upset.
- Excessive steroids can cause severe muscle soreness and edema.
- Excessive linseed oil and excessively large amounts of vitamin supplements can cause tinnitus, muscle soreness, and other problems.
- Niacin, especially above 100 milligrams, causes a niacin flush in normal people—face and ears red and tingling for a few minutes immediately after taking.

A number of patients who had been taking prescription medications for several years found that within several weeks after going on the Standard Omega-3 Program using linseed oil, a number of toxic effects occurred that were typical of the drugs. These effects invariably disappeared when the dosage of the medication was lowered, so don't always blame problems on the nutritional supplements.

Everyone who is taking prescription medication should discuss possible medication side-effects with his or her physician or check the *Physicians Desk Reference* (often available in your local library). If you take any over-the-counter (OTC) medications, be alert to changes in your total health. If any of the symptoms of drug toxicity appear after you start the Omega Supplemental Program, find out if a lowered dose of medication is feasible. If it is not, then lower the linseed oil dose.

External topical application of linseed oil

One subject in the pilot study reported that applying linseed oil topically to the skin of her varicose veins reduced the pain that had been brought on by walking. Other subjects have noticed that arthritis and eczema improved from local application of linseed oil. However, I have also seen irritations result from applying linseed oil to seborrheic dermatitis of the face and scalp. A good precaution would be to test a small, dime-sized area of skin for at least forty-eight hours.

NUTRIENTS TO EMPHASIZE IN SPECIFIC ILLNESSES

The chart that follows is my compilation, based on my general experience and research. The conclusions are not definitively established fact. If you experience severe or persistent symptoms, consult your doctor. Find your health problem; look to the right on the chart and find the nutrition supplements that may be helpful to you, but always work toward a complete, balanced Omega Supplement Program.

Nutrients That May Provide Relief from Illness

Problem or Illness	Explore the effects of these nutrients
Acne	Vitamins pro-A, A, E; folic acid, selenium, Omega-3 EFA, fiber, lactobacillus
Alcoholism	All B vitamins, vitamin E, selenium, Omega-3 EFA, fiber
Aging	Vitamins pro-A and A, all B vitamins, vitamin E, calcium, zinc, magnesium, selenium, Omega-3 EFA, fiber, lactobacillus
Anemia	Vitamin B_{12}, iron
Antisocial behavior	All B vitamins, vitamin E, zinc, magnesium, selenium, Omega-3 EFA
Arthritis	Vitamins B_2, B_3, and B_6; calcium, zinc, magnesium, selenium, Omega-3 EFA
Bruising	All B vitamins, vitamins C and E, calcium, selenium, Omega-3 EFA
Bursitis	Vitamins B_2, B_6, B_{12}, and E; calcium, magnesium, selenium, Omega-3 EFA
Cancer	Vitamins pro-A and A, all the B vitamins, vitamin E, calcium, magnesium, selenium, Omega-3 EFA, fiber, lactobacillus
Cardiovascular disease	Vitamins B_3 and E, zinc, magnesium, selenium, Omega-3 EFA, fiber
Cataracts	Vitamins pro-A, A, B_2, C, and E; folic acid, magnesium
Cystic fibrosis	Vitamin E, selenium, Omega-3 EFA
Dandruff	All B vitamins, vitamin E, magnesium, selenium, Omega-3 EFA

Problem or Illness	Explore the effects of these nutrients
Depression	Folic acid, vitamin B_6, magnesium, selenium, Omega-3 EFA, fiber, lactobacillus, chromium
Diabetes	All B vitamins, vitamin E, selenium, Omega-3 EFA, lactobacillus, chromium
Dupuytren's contracture	Vitamins B_2, B_6, and E; Omega-3 EFA
Dyspareunia	Folic acid, vitamin E, selenium, Omega-3 EFA
Endocrine problems	All B vitamins, vitamin E, selenium, Omega-3 EFA
Headache	Vitamin E, magnesium, selenium, Omega-3 EFA
Herpes	All B vitamins, calcium, zinc, 1–3 grams of lysine per day
Hypertension	All B vitamins, calcium, Omega-3 EFA
Hypotension	All B vitamins, Omega-3 EFA
Immune disorders	All B vitamins, vitamin E, selenium, Omega-3 EFA
Infertility	All B vitamins, vitamin E, selenium, Omega-3 EFA
Mastitis	All B vitamins, vitamin E, selenium, Omega-3 EFA
Menopausal problems	All B vitamins, vitamin E, calcium, selenium, Omega-3 EFA
Multiple sclerosis	All B vitamins, vitamin E, selenium, Omega-3 EFA
Nail problems	Calcium, zinc, Omega-3 EFA, thyroid supplements, protein supplements
Neuropathy	Vitamins B_1, B_{12}, and E; selenium, Omega-3 EFA
Neurosis	All B vitamins, vitamin E, selenium, Omega-3 EFA

Problem or Illness	Explore the effects of these nutrients
Obesity	All B vitamins, vitamin E, magnesium, selenium, Omega-3 EFA, chromium, fiber
Osteoporosis	Vitamin D, calcium, estrogens
Premenstrual Syndrome (PMS)	Vitamin B_6, zinc, magnesium, selenium, Omega-3 EFA
Prostatic hypertrophy	Folic acid, selenium, Omega-3 EFA, vitamin E
Psoriasis	Vitamins B_2 and B_6, zinc, magnesium, selenium, Omega-3 EFA
Psychosis	Vitamins B_1, B_3, B_6, and E; magnesium, selenium, Omega-3 EFA, fiber, lactobacillus
Raynaud's syndrome	Folic acid, vitamin E, selenium, Omega-3 EFA
High serum cholesterol	Vitamin B_3, vitamin E, selenium, Omega-3 EFA, fiber
Skin/hair problems	Vitamins pro-A, A, C, and E; folic acid, selenium, Omega-3 EFA
Taste/smell disorders	Calcium, zinc
Tinnitus	Vitamins B_1 and B_{12}, Omega-3 EFA
Trauma healing	All B vitamins, vitamin E, selenium, Omega-3 EFA
Vision	Vitamins pro-A, A, B_2, B_6, and E; selenium, Omega-3 EFA

Part III

The Omega Diets: Getting It All Together

The Omega diets provide the first comprehensive dietary regimens that consider the important Omega-3 factor—the nutritional missing link—in human nutrition.

This section includes discussions of dietary principles and food groupings, and provides a shopping guide that you can take with you to your supermarket.

Menus and recipes for the every day Standard Omega Diet, the Omega Weight Loss Program (including Omega Easy-thin, Omega Gourmet-thin, and Omega Veggie-thin diets), the Omega Anti-allergy diets, the Omega Mother-Infant Diet, and the Omega Anti-aging Diet are also provided in this section.

15

The Omega EFA and the Three Traditional Food Groups

T he Standard Omega-3 Diet is a practical balance between the ideal and the practical. It keeps you healthy, based as it is on time-tested nutritional guidelines and nutritionally innovative thinking, and deals with the existing food base. Like traditional basic diets, the Standard Omega-3 Diet classifies foods into basic groups.

FOOD GROUPS FROM THE OMEGA VIEWPOINT

The basic three food groups for every diet

We may not be able to or want to eat the same foods our ancestors ate. However, a pattern runs through all traditional diets, and no matter on which continent or in which climate they developed, they have all passed the test of time. Traditional eating patterns were based on three food groups:

Group 1. Fruits, berries, and yellow/green vegetables

Examples	Nutrients provided
Yams, apples, potatoes	Vitamins A, C, E, folic acid, minerals
Carrots, apricots	Fiber, some protein, EFA, and vitamins pro-A, A and B

Group 2. Cereals, seeds, nuts*

Examples	Nutrients provided
Wheat, rye, or oats	Vitamin E and B, minerals, and fiber
Walnuts, flaxseed, chestnuts, hazelnuts, beechnuts	Protein and EFA

*Sprouted seeds/grains are good sources of vitamin C and Omega-3 EFA. In sprouted form, some of their sugars turn into vitamin C, providing a good winter source when fruits and vegetables are scarce.

Group 3. Legumes, meats, fish, and dairy products

Examples	Nutrients provided
Lentils, lamb, bluefish, cheese	Combined with Group-2 protein sources, produce complete amino acid balances; fiber, vitamins B and E, folic acid, minerals, and EFA (fish and beans)

The three basic food groups, together with fresh water and oil from locally grown seeds or nuts, served for centuries to provide safe, satisfying, and nutritionally complete fare. They are still a good source of nutrition today. Choose the foods in each of the three basic groups that will restore a normal Omega-3/Omega-6 balance of fats in your body appropriate for your needs and your climate. (Remember, cold climates require more Omega-3.)

Adding some Omega supplements to the three food groups

Eating foods from the three basic groups at every meal should supply all the needed essential nutrients, provided you select the right ones. While following this diet, it may not be absolutely necessary to add a multimineral/multivitamin supplement that provides a minimum RDA, but it is still prudent to do so, in view of aging and eating habits. Include the following supplements in your daily diet:

- Vitamin C, 500 milligrams
- Vitamin E, 50 to 100 IU
- Calcium carbonate or calcium gluconate, 1 to 2 grams
- One spoon of flaxseed, wheat germ, linseed oil, *or* cod liver oil
- Selenium, 10 to 50 micrograms

Fruits, Vegetables, and Grains
for Omega Eaters

Fruits and vegetables are important in your diet

Eat four to six servings of yellow/green vegetables and fruits every day to meet your carotene (pro-vitamin A) needs. Some sources are:

Apricots	Chard	Squash
Beet greens	Collard greens	Sweet potatoes
Broccoli	Papaya	Tomatoes
Cantaloupe	Peaches	Watermelon
Carrots	Spinach	Yams

Each fruit or vegetable provides specific nutrient benefits. Apricots, for example, are a good source of potassium, a fighter against high blood pressure, and as a beta-carotene food defend against cancer.

Vegetables from the Sea
Contain Omega-3 and Fiber

Fresh sea vegetables—kelp, dulse, nori, and all other edible marine algae—are an excellent source of EPA, a super-polyunsaturated Omega-3 fat. Seaweeds and plankton are the only plants that contain this fatty acid. Unfortunately, the fat content of sea algae is low and disappears entirely when the plants are dried after harvesting. However, even dried, sea vegetables are valuable for their minerals and vitamins and because they provide special kinds of hydrophilic (moisture absorbing) fiber. The fibers are similar to cellulose in land plants but softer. Glucomannan is one example. Japanese scientists have noted the soothing, regulating action of these fibers in the digestive tract. Another plus for sea vegetables is that they are low in calories.

How cereals, vegetables, and fiber all work together

Observe the following guidelines in order to get the best nutrients from nonmeat products:

- Use stone ground flours, bread made from whole grains, and pastas and pastries made with stone ground flour. Use only breakfast cereals that are labeled as having more than 2 percent dietary fiber content. (Some now contain added flaxseed, as do Roman Meal–type breads.)
- Avoid refined white flours and products made from them—from breads to cakes. They offer little nutritive value. Some of these products are called "enriched," but even then they lack fiber, vitamin B_6, calcium, selenium, and EFA.
- When possible eat whole fruits without peeling or purees of the whole fruit for the benefits of the fiber and pectin. (But be sure to wash carefully and rinse completely.)
- Enjoy well-washed raw vegetables as often as possible. Make them part of your snacks, garnishes, and salads.
- Reduce the cooking time of cooked vegetables. Boiled, steamed, or sautéed vegetables should be slightly crisp when served, unless you have ulcerative colitis.
- Use fresh or frozen vegetables instead of canned vegetables. (This provides the fiber and avoids the sugar and salt in most canned foods.) If you do use canned vegetables, make sure they are salt-free.

• Take a premeal fiber supplement before each meal. (See page 29 for the recipe.)

Northern Nuts and Seeds

Nuts and seeds are high in unsaturated fatty acids. They provide vitamin E, folic acid, protein, and minerals such as magnesium to your diet. They also have a crisp texture that makes them ideal garnishes and side dishes. If you eat nuts, know what you're eating, so you can balance your intake of Omega-3 and Omega-6 EFA.

Nuts

Chestnuts, beechnuts, walnuts, and hazelnuts are rich in Omega-3 and Omega-6. Select northern nuts over southern-grown nuts such as peanuts (not actually a nut, but a legume) and cashews.

Northern Nuts	Southern Nuts
Walnuts	Peanuts
Hazelnuts	Cashews
Beechnuts	Pecans
Chestnuts	Brazil nuts

Seeds

Pumpkin, sunflower, sesame, and other seeds are high in oil content and high in calories. Flaxseed is very high in Omega-3 EFA and was eaten in ancient Rome as a nutty condiment.

Seeds are best used in small amounts. Eat no more than one ounce of seeds (a large handful) a day. Seeds are delightful flavor enhancers when added to main dishes, and you can blend seeds with legumes and vegetables to contribute the valuable proteins, vitamin E, EFA, and minerals (such as potassium and magnesium) needed for a healthful diet.

Legumes

Northern beans

Nutritionally complete single-dish meals (see pages 152–156) will provide the RDA for Omega-3 and Omega-6 EFA even before salad or cooking oil is added. When possible use cold-climate beans (navy, common, red, and kidney), as these have more Omega-3 EFA than southern-grown varieties.

Fortify the northern beans with one teaspoon of walnut, soybean, or linseed oil, if only to cover any deficit created by a lifetime of low or marginal EFA intake. Northern beans include:

Common beans	Pinto beans	Soybeans
Kidney beans	Red beans	Yankee beans
Navy beans		

These northern beans supply a greater proportion of Omega-3 EFA than Omega-6 EFA. Soybeans, an outstanding source of Omega-3 and fiber, are a complete protein as well, containing all the essential amino acids in the optimum combination and amounts. All other legumes— black-eyed peas, black beans, mung beans, garbanzo beans, green peas, lentils, and peanuts—are still valuable foods, despite their low Omega-3 value, because of their high nutrient (e.g., folic acid) and fiber content but need the protein of cereal grains or nuts to be complete. All legumes are normalizers of blood sugars in non–insulin-dependent diabetes.

Gas-Free Beans

Utah State University's nutrition department has found an easy way to reduce the tendency for flatulence that prevents many people from enjoying beans. Sprouting is the secret.

The gas producers are complex sugars stored within dry beans, which our intestinal enzymes cannot digest. But when a bean starts to germinate, it quickly breaks down the complex sugars into simple ones, which are then used for energy by the rapidly growing seedlings. After about two to four days of germination, almost all of the offending sugars—and the gas they produce— have disappeared.

Easy Bean Sprouting

1. Rinse enough beans for one or two meals and place in a jar.
2. Add spring or bottled water to cover.
3. Allow the beans to soak for five to six hours at room temperature.
4. Drain water, and rinse gently with cold water twice daily.
5. Keep the jar in a warm place to speed germination.
6. Watch for tiny white rootlets to appear in two to four days.
7. When you see rootlets the beans are ready for cooking or baking.

Another way to reduce gas potential is just to soak the beans overnight in five parts of water and change the water two or three times. When soaked and pressure cooked to tenderness, the beans will cause little digestive trouble.

In *Diet for a Small Planet,* Frances Moore Lappe describes the protein-supplying dishes of most traditional diets as consisting of one part legumes plus two to four parts cereals. The result is a satisfying meal. This ratio produces food that provides all the essential amino acids in the correct proportions needed by the human body—it delivers complete protein. (The one-dish meals given later employ this ratio.) However, eggs, milk, soybeans, meat, and fish are complete proteins in themselves. Supplements of egg, milk, or soybean protein are filling and can help you to lose weight. Interestingly, they also seem to reduce fingernail blemishes and other nail problems, especially when supplemented with zinc.

Meats and Fish

Before modern times, few but the rich could afford to eat meat or fowl on a regular basis. For most people, the daily fare was whole-grain cereals, coarse bread, legumes, potatoes, vegetables, and fruit. Chestnut bread, called "tree bread," was common and high in Omega-3. The high-fiber/mineral/EFA/vitamin foods protected people from the kinds of problems that arise from high-fat flesh or dairy foods. The same dietary focus will have that effect today.

While I think the average modern diet contains too much meat, I do not recommend a vegetarian diet. The use of Group 2 foods plus Group 3 legumes to provide complete protein should at least be supplemented by fish several times a week (one to two pounds) to create an ideal diet. Meats can be used as a garnish or reserved for a main dish once or twice a week.

Beef—low in Omega EFA

Use beef sparingly. It is low in Omega EFA. Avoid marbled beef. Do not use any smoked or prepared "luncheon meats" or sausage, because these products are high in saturated fats, nitrates, and sodium. *Even the new lower-fat "chicken franks" should be avoided because they are still very high in saturated fat, sodium, and nitrates.*

Organ meats like liver, kidney, and heart contain Omega-6 fatty acid. Sweetbread (thymus) is too high in saturated fats. An occasional meal of liver, heart, or kidney is a good idea because of their rich supply of folic acid, B vitamins, and other nutrients.

Pork—most is low-Omega EFA

Pork that comes from swine fed on a traditional livestock diet of grains and legumes will be high in Omega-3 and Omega-6 EFA and you can eat it normally. Most commercial pork, however, is now fed corn, a low EFA source, so should be eaten sparingly. If you must have a treat of bacon for breakfast one or two times a week, use the new lean or "gourmet" bacon cuts, e.g., "Canadian bacon."

Lamb—also low in Omega EFA

Lamb is not high in Omega EFA because, like cows, sheep are ruminants, and ruminant bacteria destroy Omega EFA. Should you decide to include it in your diet occasionally, roast or broil cuts that have been carefully trimmed of fat.

Fowl—low-fat is best

The wild game and fowl (as well as small animals such as rabbit) that early man enjoyed were lean and the flesh contained a much higher proportion of stringy muscle and unsaturated fats than does the modern domesticated chicken. The modern, plump birds are delicious because of all the fat oozing through their flesh—but the fat should be avoided. Favor low-fat chicken (breasts without skin) for an occasional treat.

High-Omega fish—dark and torpedo shaped

Fish and other seafood, besides containing minerals, and high quality protein, are the best sources of EPA and DHA. These Omega-3 fatty acids are essential to eyes, brain, and arteries, as well as testes, although the body can in most cases make these fatty acids from plant Omega-3 EFA (alpha linolenic acid).

To increase your intake of super-polyunsaturated Omega-3 EPA and DHA, eat dark, cold-water, fatty fish such as:

Albacore tuna	Herring	Russian sturgeon
American eel	Mackerel	Salmon
Anchovies	Pilchard	Sardines
Bluefish	Rainbow trout	Sprat

The fat that comes from these fish is the kind of fat that helps the heart and arteries—a "good" fat. Even the leanest of those listed contain some EPA and DHA.

Flat, white fish generally contain little EFA, although what they do contain is Omega-3 in type. This is because these flat fish are reef or bottom dwellers designed for short bursts of maneuverable swimming. Dark fish are usually torpedo-shaped and designed for long distance swimming, so they store lots of EFA and fat, making the meat dark.

Dairy Products and Omega Power

Cheese, yogurt, milk, buttermilk, and butter—from cows, goats, sheep, mares, and/or reindeer—are staples in many diets. But note: Except for mares and reindeer, all are ruminants whose digestive systems destroy the EFA. Only mare and reindeer meat and milk are high in EFA, especially Omega-3 EFA. However, all soured or cultured milk products are good sources of *lactobacillus acidophilus* and other friendly lactic acid bacteria.

Special warnings about milk and milk products

Once human beings pass early childhood, many no longer make the intestinal enzyme lactase, which is needed to digest milk sugar (lactose). Lactose is plentiful in fresh milk and fresh milk products.

If you suffer from diarrhea, excess gas, or bloating after eating a milk product, you may be one of those who have a lactase deficiency. You should then switch from whole milk products to a new specially treated milk recently marketed for the lactase deficient, or to cheese, yogurt, and soured milk. The lactose content in sour milk products is lower than in fresh milk. Bacteria in cultured products help to break down the lactose.

If you cannot tolerate any dairy products, you can still obtain all the nutrients you need from the basic Group 1, 2, and 3 foods without milk products.

Making bacteria work for you

The beneficial (aerobic) bacteria we want to populate our intestinal tract depend on:

- Dietary fiber to provide the right growth medium
- Antibodies in the digestive tract
- Direct seeding from oral intake (cheeses and yogurt)

Eating yogurt and cheese can often introduce needed bacteria into the digestive system. Use low-sugar yogurt as part of a premeal mixed fiber–yogurt cocktail. Even if the milk in the yogurt is pasteurized, the yogurt itself is usually not pasteurized, so that it contains living, useful bacteria of the *lactobacillus* group. However, watch out. Some producers now also pasteurize the yogurt itself to extend shelf life while destroying its benefits, just as steel roller milling extends the shelf life of cereal products while destroying fiber, vitamins, and EFA and just as hydrogenation extends oil shelf life while destroying EFA. NOTE: Helpful *lactobacillus acidophilus* bacteria are available in powder or capsules without milk as a base.

GENERAL RULES
FOR OMEGAFYING YOUR DIET

The Standard Omega Diet will benefit everyone, whether by itself or as part of the Omega supplemental (therapeutic) regimen for specific ailments. (See Part II.) It is designed to keep and enhance your health.

Normalize your intake of oils and essential fats

Everyone benefits from the following ways of normalizing EFA intake:

• Try to use no more than one to two pats of butter a day, because butter is high in saturated fat.
• All oils should be Omega-3 cold-pressed liquid oils (soy, walnut, linseed, or wheat germ). Use no hydrogenated oils or margarine. While olive or sesame oil are good substitutes for the saturated fat of meat, they do not contain much EFA.

A Viking's daily diet would have supplied the amount of Omega-3 EFA provided in about two teaspoons of linseed oil a day, if the Viking ate a daily total of about 2,000 calories. Modern diets supply no more than the equivalent of one-quarter teaspoon of the Omega-3 in linseed oil, or one-eighth of the amount in a traditional diet.

Additionally, saturated and hydrogenated fats increase our Omega-3 EFA requirements. Therefore, as a safety measure, I suggest taking one teaspoon of flaxseed, linseed oil, or cod liver oil daily. I also suggest taking a one-a-day multivitamin and multimineral supplement that includes the antioxidants vitamin pro-A, C, E, and selenium. Finally, routinely take the premeal fiber cocktail "appetizer."

Add Omega oils to your diet

Cooking, baking, or light sautéing does not destroy the essential fatty acids in linseed oil. However, do not use linseed oil in high temperature frying, because it tends to smoke. Use linseed oil in salads, vinaigrettes, marinades, and for dressings whenever a food oil is needed (see recipes).

Some people don't like the flavor of linseed oil. While some describe it as "nutty," other find it "fishy." If that is your reaction, use soy or walnut oil or a mixture of either of these oils together or with linseed oil. Buy oils in pint quantities and refrigerate after unsealing them. Discard any oil if you detect the slightest rancid odor or taste.

Oils must be used sparingly because they have a high caloric content—about 110 calories per tablespoon—and because they tend to increase the body's requirements for selenium and vitamin E. **Caution:** *Never use paint-base linseed oil. It has been chemically modified and is dangerous.*

Keep sugar out of your diet

Six of the forty-four subjects in the pilot study group reported markedly bad effects from consuming sugar. The reactions ranged from feelings of malaise within an hour after eating high-sugar products to aggravation of the symptoms of their particular illnesses. These symptoms included tinnitus, feelings of severe anxiety, and even psychosis.

Refined sugar is more a drug than a food; it disturbs the metabolic system. Even when you receive no immediate body signals, sugar is affecting you adversely. You should avoid or use it as sparingly as possible. Sugar products offer only calories without any of the vitamins and minerals the body requires to process foods. These are properly called "empty calories," meaning they come without the essential nutrients required to metabolize them and thus contribute to what is called an "induced deficiency."

Omega Antifreeze

Winter wheat, like other cold-climate plants, is cold-resistant because it produces large amounts of Omega-3 EFA in response to cold weather. This Omega-3 prevents its cell membranes from freezing and fracturing. Cold-climate plants also produce large amounts of a sugarlike water-soluble material called glycerol, which prevents their watery fluids from freezing in cold weather. Cold-resistant plants produce proportionately more Omega-3 EFA than Omega-6. We can think of Omega-3 as a sort of winterizing oil, and Omega-6 as a sort of summerizing oil.

Animals and man must ultimately get their EFA directly from plants or indirectly via plant-eating animals. Temperate and cold-climate dwelling animals are normally supplied with large amounts of Omega-3 in their cold-climate diets. They have evolved Omega-3 EFA utilization mechanisms to control their adaptation to cold. These oils play a role in regulating hair production, skin color, fat distribution, calorie burn-off (thermogenesis) and offer protection against the cardiovascular and other damage that might be produced by the typical high-energy high-fat diet in cold climates.

Less Omega-3 is produced in warm climates than in cold climates, and less is needed by warm-climate animals and people. This natural balance of Omega-3 and Omega-6 can be disrupted either by transporting oils, plants, or people out of their normal climate zones or by destroying Omega-3 with hydrogenation. When that happens, trouble soon follows; the genetically most sensitive are the first to suffer, each person succumbing in his or her own illness pattern.

Soft drinks rob the body of its own B-vitamin, mineral, fiber, and EFA stores. The astonishing nine teaspoons of sugar in an average bottle of soda pop will leave the body nutrients depleted. Diet soft drinks are better, but many consumers become adversely sensitized to the artificial sweeteners. Prior to the nineteenth century, people ate an average of 15 pounds of sugar a year. Today sugar consumption hovers around 128 pounds per capita per year, nearly a 1,000 percent increase. In my experience, every patient who reduced sugar intake to a minimum enjoyed substantial health rewards.

Make sure that you get enough water

Drink only water that has been stored in glass (never plastic) containers. Drink at least one eight-ounce glass with each premeal fiber cocktail. This alone will amount to three glasses daily. Then drink at least three additional glasses of water. Water is especially important if you suffer from constipation or irritable bowel syndrome.

City water is usually acceptable for cooking, but in several studies with primates, bowel and bladder cancer have been linked to drinking heavily chlorinated water, and there is growing concern about lead entering from solder joints. Until similar studies are completed on the effects of another water additive, fluoride, its safety is still in question. If you live in a community that does not have fluoridated water, it is preferable to use fluoride toothpaste to prevent dental cavities than to introduce fluorides into the water supply.

16
The Omega Shopping Guide

The first step in any diet is a trip to the supermarket or health food store. If you're going to change your food pattern, start with your food shopping.

Supermarket shopping

The supermarket is a nutritional minefield because about 80 percent of our food is processed and imported from other climates. That 80 percent is:

Acidified
Antibiotically treated
Antioxidated
Artificially colored
Artificially flavored
Broiled-boiled
Bromated
Chlorinated
Defatted
Defibered
Degerminated
Dehydrated

Emulsified
Enriched by chemical means
Fried
Hybridized
Hydrogenated
Marbled
Nitrated
Phosphated
Salted
Sugared
Supplemented artificially

The collective effects of these modifications have never been determined by scientific tests.

Your goal is to correct the loss of essential nutrients as a result of processing and to avoid the introduced antinutrients. You want to make the food you eat at least 70 percent nutritionally active.

The ideal goal is to eat what A. Hoffer, a leader in nutritional science, calls "live food." By this he means traditional fresh food with nothing added and nothing removed—foods that are indigenously grown. We do not actually know the nutritive value of many modern hybrid plants grown by modern farming methods. For example, some agriculturists and veterinarians are concerned about a selenium deficiency in food grown outside the Midwest.

It is important to check labels on products

When reading labels, notice which ingredients appear first on the list. Those that appear first are there in the highest proportion. Look for Omega oils (nonhydrogenated soy, walnut, wheat germ) and stone-ground and whole grains to be prominent in any list. Reject products that include high proportions of saturated fats, sugars, salt, and refined flours. Too often food processors add sugar and salt to encourage you to eat more than you should.

Read Labels

Favor	Reduce
Cold-pressed plant or fish oils	Hydrogenated oils and tallows
Nonhydrogenated oils	Margarine
Low saturated fats	Partially hydrogenated oils
High Omega-3 polyunsaturates	Southern oils and nuts
Whole grains	Saturated fats
Stone-ground whole flour	Beef and lamb
Fiber content of 2% or more	Defatted grains
Breads from stone-ground grains	Instant cereals
Pastas from stone-ground grains	Refined sugar or corn syrup
Fresh, dark fish	Refined flour
Cold-climate beans, cereals, and nuts	Pastas/breads from refined flours (groats and grits)
Whole-grain, unsweetened cereals	Low-fiber prepared foods
	High salt-content foods
	Preservatives
	Artificial coloring and flavors
	Nitrates and nitrites

Making Food Choices
Produce

Favor	Reduce
In-season	Out-of-season
Local	Imported or exotic
Fresh	Canned or frozen (but frozen is better than canned)
Unprocessed	Processed

Fish, Fowl, Meat, and Legumes

Favor	Reduce (to no more than 8 oz. per week)
Fresh fish (but dark fish—e.g., tuna, salmon, mackerel, herring, trout, bluefish—over white, flat fish	Beef
	Lamb
	Pork from commercially fed swine
Fish canned with water or, even better, in natural fish oil	Fish canned with hydrogenated vegetable oil
Chicken, duck, game birds	Cold cuts, sausages, or hot dogs
Meat from nonruminant wild animals (e.g., venison)	
Pork from properly fed swine	
Navy, common, red, northern, and pinto beans	

Dairy

Favor	Reduce
Milk, skim or protein-fortified	Chocolate milk
Yogurt	Margarine
Butter (but use sparingly)	
Cheeses (but use sparingly)	

Cooking and Salad Oils

Favor	Avoid
Soy	Safflower
Walnut	Peanut
Wheat germ	Corn
Linseed	Cottonseed
Olive (in moderation)	Coconut
	Palm kernel

Drinks

Favor	Avoid
Fruit purees	Fruit juices (no fiber)
Milk, skim and protein-fortified	Sugared and caffeinated soft drinks
Water-decaffeinated coffee and tea	Coffee and tea

Desserts

Favor	Reduce
Fruits	Ice cream
Granola bars	Candy
Nuts (northern)	Cakes, pies, and pastries
Applesauce	containing refined sugar
Cheeses (but use sparingly)	

Stocking Your Pantry

Oils (cold-pressed)
Soybean
Walnut
Wheat germ
Linseed

Cereal Grains
Whole wheat,
  northern
Whole buckwheat
Whole bulgur wheat
Whole rye
Whole oats
Brown rice
Corn (use sparingly)
Whole barley
Whole millet

Peas and Beans
  (legumes)
Dried peas
Dried lentils
Dried beans,
  northern type: soy,
  black, garbanzo,
  kidney, navy, red,
  pinto

Flours
Stone-ground whole
  wheat
Stone-ground
  chestnut
Stone-ground
  soybean powder
Stone-ground corn
  (use sparingly)

Nuts
Walnuts
Chestnuts
Hazelnuts
Beechnuts

Prepared Cereals (at
  least 2% crude
  fiber)
Wheat germ
40% bran and all-
  bran flakes (try the
  Uncle Sam brand,
  which has flaxseed
  added)
Raisin bran
Grape Nuts
Shredded Wheat

Seeds
Flaxseed (use no
  more than 1–2
  teaspoons daily)
Chia seeds
Pumpkin seeds
Sunflower (use no
  more than 1 ounce
  daily)

Fiber
Miller's bran
Psyllium seed
Apple pectin
Glucomannan

Pastas (made with
  stone-ground flour
  if possible)
Shells
Flat noodles
Bow ties
Spirals
Linguine
Spaghetti
Elbow macaroni
Spinach noodles

Condiments
Worcestershire sauce
Prepared mustard
Catsup
Black olives
Green olives
Soy sauce
Mayonnaise (made
  with cold-pressed
  soy oil)*
Tabasco sauce

Fresh Vegetables
  (as wide a variety as
  your local super-
  market can
  supply—favor local
  varieties)
Artichokes
Asparagus
Bamboo shoots
Beet greens
Beets
Broccoli
Brussels sprouts

Cabbage
Carrots
Cauliflower
Celery
Chard
Collard greens
Cucumber
Dandelion greens
Eggplant
Endive
Escarole
Kale
Lettuce
Leeks
Mung bean sprouts
Mushrooms
Mustard greens
Okra
Onions
Oyster plant
Parsley
Parsnips
Peas
Peppers
Potatoes
Pumpkin
Radishes
Rutabagas
Spinach
Scallions
Squash (winter)
String beans
Summer squash
Tomatoes
Turnips
Turnip greens
Watercress

*Hain's is a brand name sold in many health food stores. The manufacturer also produces a mayonnaise made with cold-pressed nonhydrogenated soy oil.

Fresh Fruits
Apples
Apricots
Grapefruit
Grapes
Melons
Oranges
Pears
Peaches
Plums
Prunes
Raisins
Other locally grown
    fruits

Dairy
Butter
Buttermilk
Cheeses (favor low-fat)
    Cheddar
    Cream
    Gouda
    Gruyère
    Cottage
Eggs (no more than 2
    per week)
Milk
Sour cream
Yogurt (low-fat, low-
    sugar)

17

The Nutritionally Complete Everyday Omega Diet

I am convinced that the nutritionally complete everyday Omega Diet can prevent many, if not most, of our illnesses.

Advantages of the Omega diet in comparison with others

Medically based. All of the Omega diets are similar to those recommended by the medical profession; they supply all needed nutrients for good health. However, I have further ensured that Omega-3 fatty acids and sufficient fiber are in every menu and every recipe. This makes the Omega Diet the first nutritionally complete diet.

Flexible and easy to use. All the Omega diets (the Everyday Standard Omega Diet and the specialized Omega diets given later in this book) can be used alone or combined with the Omega Supplement Program.

Exercise-linked. The Omega diets and the Omega Supplement Program will be helpful to everyone, but all diets should be integrated with reasonable exercise programs for the optimum effects. Exercise and nutrition are mutually reinforcing. Stress reduction also contributes to the beneficial effects to be gained.

Therapeutically beneficial. Finally, the Omega diets can be used to enhance the nutritional content and augment the potential for success of any therapeutic diet designed to help those suffering from drug abuse or alcoholism. They also work with anti-smoking and weight loss programs and act to reinforce many treatments for trauma and for chronic diseases.

THE STANDARD OMEGA DIET—AN OVERVIEW

Summary of the general rules for Omega eating

The menus developed and tested for the nutritionally complete Standard Omega Diet adhere to the important principles discussed in Part I. A complete week of menus is provided. You can scale the menus up to gourmet level or down to simple country fare. You can be as extravagant or as frugal as your tastes and your budget decree. However, you must adhere to the following guidelines for the best results. (You will note these echo the food choice recommendations given in the preceding chapter on shopping.)

- Reduce red meat consumption to one to two servings per week. Increase chicken and have a minimum of two fish meals per week (at least one pound), preferably dark fish (e.g., tuna, mackerel, bluefish, rock fish, herring, salmon).
- Reduce sugar. Try fructose or use a sugar substitute if necessary.
- Eliminate caffeine (one cup of coffee or tea for breakfast, only if you must). Use water-decaffeinated coffee or decaffeinated tea, and be wary of caffeine in other drinks or foods. Here is a list of the milligrams of caffeine per average serving of various drinks:

Coffee (automatic drip)	181
Tea (strong)	90
Tea (English breakfast)	107
Dr. Pepper	38
Cocoa	45

- Avoid margarine and hydrogenated or southern oils. Use butter sparingly.
- Use only nonhydrogenated soybean, walnut, wheat germ, or linseed oils for cooking and salads. Use only mayonnaise made from nonhydrogenated oils.
- Eat walnuts, chestnuts, hazelnuts, beechnuts; avoid other nuts.
- Add small amounts of seeds—e.g., sunflower or flaxseed—to your foods, or eat them as a snack.
- Use whole fruits or purees of whole fruit, not the juices.
- Cook vegetables lightly and serve when still slightly crisp *(al dente)*.
- Use a few teaspoons of wheat germ for breakfast cereal, and eat only cereals containing more than 2 percent dietary fiber (All-Bran, 40% Bran Flakes, Shredded Wheat, and Uncle Sam are examples).
- Restrict alcohol to no more than two ounces of hard liquor or four ounces of wine a day for at least two to four months; try not to drink every day.

- Adjust the proportion of meat, fish, and fowl relative to vegetables and fruits to find what makes you feel best. This must be done over a period of weeks. Be aware of changes in your skin, mood, and general stamina. If your body reacts well, continue the program.
- If your body reacts badly—if you suffer any unusual or unpleasant sensations—to any food, then reduce the intake of that food and replace it with an alternative of approximately equivalent nutritional value.
- Eat and drink slowly to give the sensation of fullness time to build (about twenty minutes is needed for your brain to know your stomach is full). Never overeat. Stop at the first sign of fullness.
- For snacks, rely on raw vegetables such as celery or carrot sticks (see snack list in this book and post it in the kitchen).
- Drink water often, especially when hungry.
- Avoid eating bread and butter before dinner.

Your minimum daily requirements

The following chart provides a listing of the nutrients necessary for adequate nutrition. This chart was worked out over decades. The menus for the Standard Diet (given later in this chapter) provide all of these required nutrients.

Recommended Daily Allowances (RDA) for the Essential Nutrients in the Approximate Complete Adult Standard Diet (2,500 Calories)

Nutrient	Standard RDA	Upper Limit	Nutrient	Standard RDA	Upper Limit
Water	700 cc.	3 liters	*Water-soluble vitamins*		
			B₁ (thiamine)	2.0 mg.	200 mg.
Bulk minerals			B₂ (riboflavin)	2.0 mg.	200 mg.
Sodium	2.0 gm.	40.0 gm.	B₃ (niacin)	20.0 mg.	3.0 gm.
Potassium	4.0 gm.	20.0 gm.	B₅ (pantothenic		
Calcium	1.0 gm.	3.0 gm.	acid)	10.0 mg.	1.0 gm.
Phosphorus	1.0 gm.	2.0 gm.	B₆ (pyridoxine)	2.0 mg.	0.5 gm.
Magnesium	0.4 gm.	2.0 gm.	B₁₂		
			(cyanocobalamin)	5.0 mcg.	1.0 mg.
Trace minerals (Non-chelates)			Folic acid (folate)	0.5 mg.	2.0 mg.
Iron	15.0 mg.	200 mg.	Biotin	0.1 mg.	0.5 mg.
Zinc	15.0 mg.	200 mg.	C (ascorbate)	50.0 mg.	10.0 gm.
Manganese	4.0 mg.	20 mg.			
Copper	2.0 mg.	20 mg.	*Oil-soluble vitamins*		
Fluoride	2.0 mg.	20 mg.	A (retinol)	5,000.0 IU	50,000 IU
Molybdenum	0.4 mg.	4 mg.	D (calciferol)	500.0 IU	1,000 IU
Iodine	0.2 mg.	2.0 mg.	E (tocopherol)	50.0 IU	1,000 IU
Selenium	0.2 mg.	0.5 mg.	K (menadione)	0.5 mg.	
Chromium	0.1 mg.	0.5 mg.			

where B₁ is B_1, B₂ is B_2, B₃ is B_3, B₅ is B_5, B₆ is B_6, B₁₂ is B_{12}.

Nutrient	Standard RDA	Upper Limit	Nutrient	Standard RDA	Upper Limit
Amino acids (approximate)†			*Fiber*	30 gm.	
Arginine	1.0 gm.		*As daily supplement:*		
Histidine	1.0 gm.		Bran (miller's)	3 Tbsp. (12 gm.)	6 Tbsp.
Isoleucine	1.0 gm.		Pectin	1 tsp. (12 gm.)	6 tsp.
Leucine	1.0 gm.		Psyllium seed	1 tsp. (12 gm.)	6 tsp.
Lysine	1.0 gm.		Lactobacillus	Trace	?
Methionine	1.0 gm.				
Phenylalanine	1.0 gm.		*Calories* (Kg/day)	35	
Threonine	0.5 gm.				
Tryptophan	0.2 gm.				
Valine	1.0 gm.				
Fatty acids					
Linoleic (ω6)	5–10% cal.	30%			
Alpha linolenic	cal.				
(ω3)	2%	15%			

*References:
Harrison's Principles of Internal Medicine, 9th ed., (p. 400)
NAS/NRC Recommended Dietary Allowances, 9th ed., 1980
E. J. Underwood, *Trace Elements,* 4th ed., Academic Press, 1977
R. S. Goodhart and M. E. Shils, *Modern Nutrition in Health and Disease,* 6th ed., Lea & Febiger, 1980
General Nutrition Catalogue, 1981
†No upper limit has been established for amino acids.

Recommended Daily Allowances (RDA) for Fat, Protein, and Carbohydrate

The recommendations that follow are consistent with the recommendations of the American Heart Association and the American Cancer Society but go considerably beyond them.

For the ideal proportion of foods, keep:

- Carbohydrate to about 50 percent of total calories
- Fats to about 30 percent of total calories
- Protein to about 15 to 20 percent of total calories

Carbohydrates should be complex and not refined (sugars), and they should include at least 25 grams per day of dietary fiber. Rely on:

- Cereals for about 75 percent of your fiber intake
- Fruits and vegetables for about 25 percent of your fiber intake

Limit alcoholic beverages to fewer than two a day, and avoid drinking alcoholic beverages every day.

Protein should be complete either in itself, as in eggs, milk, meat, and soybeans, or made complete by mixing one part legumes (beans) to about two parts of cereal or other nonleguminous vegetable protein. The amino acid composition of these two families complement one another.

Fat should be supplied in the following way:

- Omega-3 (fish or plant), 2 to 3 percent of total calories
- Omega-6, 5 to 10 percent
- Omega-9 (monounsaturated—high, for example, in olive oil), 10 to 20 percent
- Saturated fats, as in beef and fast foods cooked in tallow, 10 percent or less

Avoid margarines, hydrogenated oils, most cold cuts, and frankfurters. Keep cholesterol to less than 100 milligrams per 1,000 calories, and avoid coconut and palm kernel oil, which are high in saturated fat.

THE STANDARD OMEGA WEEKLY MENU

The Standard Omega Diet, which is a nutritionally complete diet, uses high-Omega food products. Here is a week of typical menus. Recipes for many of the dishes are provided in the section immediately following the weekly menus. (You may substitute one of your old favorite meals occasionally.)

When using menus and following recipes:

- Always drink one glass of water with fiber.
- All oils should be nonhydrogenated, cold-pressed "Omega oils"— soy, linseed, walnut, or wheat germ oil.
- If desired, use decaffeinated coffee or decaffeinated tea, preferably black, with fructose.
- Fish may be bluefish, tuna, salmon, mackerel, trout, striped bass, swordfish, or halibut.
- To help suppress your appetite, drink a glass of water or eat celery, lettuce, carrots (one per day), cucumbers, or other raw green vegetable.
- Many recipes require a blender; if none is available, use a high-speed beater.

SUNDAY

		Calories
BREAKFAST	2–4 tablespoons fiber appetizer*	50
	½ grapefruit	40
	1½ cup 40% Bran Flakes	200
	1 slice stone-ground whole-wheat bread	75
	¾ cup skim milk	70
	1 teaspoon butter or oil	35
	TOTAL	470
LUNCH	2–4 tablespoons fiber appetizer*	50
	3 ounces skinned lean chicken (boiled, baked, or broiled)	115
	1 slice stone-ground whole-wheat bread	75
	1 teaspoon butter or oil	35
	2 cups tomato and lettuce salad	50
	1 tablespoon Omega mayonnaise**	100
	¾ cup skim milk	90
	TOTAL	515
MIDAFTERNOON SNACK	1 apple	70
	1 cup skim milk	120
	TOTAL	190
DINNER	2–4 tablespoons fiber appetizer*	50
	6 ounces bluefish (broil, serve with lemon)**	220
	½ cup carrots (raw or boiled)	35
	½ cup broccoli (boiled)	25
	2 cups tomato and lettuce salad	50
	1 tablespoon Omega mayonnaise**	100
	¼ cup chestnuts or walnuts	180
	TOTAL	660
EVENING SNACK	½ ounce low-fat cheese	40
	½ cup skim milk	60
	TOTAL	100
	GRAND TOTAL	1935

*Recipe for fiber appetizer cocktail appears on page 29.
**Recipe appears in recipe sections following these menus.

MONDAY

		Calories
BREAKFAST	2–4 tablespoons fiber appetizer*	50
	1 orange	60
	1 egg, scrambled	115
	1 slice stone-ground whole-wheat bread	75
	¾ cup skim milk	90
	1 teaspoon butter or oil	35
	TOTAL	425
LUNCH	2–4 tablespoons fiber appetizer*	50
	5 ounces tuna	175
	1 slice stone-ground whole-wheat bread	75
	1 teaspoon butter or oil	35
	2 cups tomato and lettuce salad	50
	1 tablespoon Omega mayonnaise**	100
	¾ cup skim milk	90
	TOTAL	575
MIDAFTERNOON SNACK	1 small pear	50
	5 walnuts	120
	TOTAL	170
DINNER	2–4 tablespoons fiber appetizer*	50
	4½ ounces lean beef or pork	270
	½ cup peas	60
	4 ounces boiled cabbage	10
	2 cups tomato and lettuce salad	50
	1 tablespoon Omega mayonnaise**	100
	4" wedge honeydew melon with scoop of sherbet	200
	TOTAL	740
EVENING SNACK	Cottage cheese mousse†	50
	1 cup skim milk	120
	TOTAL	170
	GRAND TOTAL	2080

*Recipe for fiber appetizer cocktail appears on page 29.
**Recipe appears in recipe sections following these menus.
†See recipe on page 206.

TUESDAY

Calories

BREAKFAST	2–4 tablespoons fiber appetizer*	50
	½ medium grapefruit, sectioned	40
	¼ cup wheat germ on	110
	1 cup shredded wheat	180
	¾ cup skim milk	90
	TOTAL	470
LUNCH	2–4 tablespoons fiber appetizer*	50
	6 ounces mackerel fillets (canned, drained)	300
	2 cups tomato and lettuce salad	50
	2 tablespoons lemon juice	10
	¾ cup skim milk	90
	TOTAL	500
MIDAFTERNOON	5 walnuts	120
SNACK	8 halves dried apricot	70
	TOTAL	190
DINNER	2–4 tablespoons fiber appetizer*	50
	6 ounces Cornish hen (roasted or broiled)	325
	½ cup beets (boiled)	30
	½ cup cauliflower (raw or steamed)	15
	(Salad and dressing optional)	(add 150)
	½ cup berries with ½ cup sherbet	190
	TOTAL	610
EVENING SNACK	1 ounce low-fat cheese	80
	½ cup skim milk	60
	TOTAL	140
	GRAND TOTAL	1910

*Recipe for fiber appetizer cocktail appears on page 29.

WEDNESDAY

		Calories
BREAKFAST	2–4 tablespoons fiber appetizer*	50
	1 medium orange, sectioned	60
	1 cup oatmeal (cooked)	130
	1 slice stone-ground whole-wheat bread	75
	1 teaspoon butter or oil	35
	¾ cup skim milk	90
	TOTAL	440
LUNCH	2–4 tablespoons fiber appetizer*	50
	1 slice stone-ground whole-wheat bread	75
	1 teaspoon butter or oil	35
	1 cup low-fat cottage cheese	180
	2 cups tomato and lettuce salad	30
	1 tablespoon Omega salad dressing	100
	¾ cup skim milk	90
	TOTAL	560
MIDAFTERNOON SNACK	15 hazelnuts	150
	20 grapes	70
	TOTAL	220
DINNER	2–4 tablespoons fiber appetizer*	50
	6 ounces lean ham or lamb (roasted)	330
	½ cup broccoli (raw or steamed)	30
	½ cup mushrooms (sautéed in oil)	40
	(Salad and dressing optional)	(add 150)
	1 apple and 1 ounce cheese	180
	TOTAL	630
EVENING SNACK	3 walnuts	70
	½ cup skim milk	60
	TOTAL	130
	GRAND TOTAL	1980

*Recipe for fiber appetizer cocktail appears on page 29.

THURSDAY

			Calories
BREAKFAST	2–4 tablespoons fiber appetizer*		50
	½ grapefruit		40
	1½ cup 40% Bran Flakes		200
	1 slice (1 oz.) lean breakfast ham		70
	¾ cup skim milk		90
	1 teaspoon butter or oil		35
		TOTAL	485
LUNCH	2–4 tablespoons fiber appetizer*		50
	4½ ounces water packed tuna		160
	¼ cup chopped scallions		10
	1 cup shredded iceburg lettuce		10
	1½ cup tomato slices and celery		30
	1 tablespoon Omega mayonnaise**		100
	1 slice bread with 1 teaspoon butter		110
	¾ cup skim milk		90
		TOTAL	560
MIDAFTERNOON SNACK	5 walnuts		120
	1 cup tomato juice		20
		TOTAL	140
DINNER	2–4 tablespoons fiber appetizer*		50
	5 ounces lamb chops (broiled)		300
	½ baked potato		70
	½ cup brussels sprouts		30
	½ cup berries with ½ cup sherbet		190
		TOTAL	640
EVENING SNACK	5 halves dried apricots		40
	1 cup plain yogurt		120
		TOTAL	160
		GRAND TOTAL	1985

*Recipe for fiber appetizer cocktail appears on page 29.
**Recipe appears in recipe sections following these menus.

FRIDAY

		Calories
BREAKFAST	2–4 tablespoons fiber appetizer*	50
	2–3 dried prunes	50
	2 pancakes (5″ × ½″), made with stone-ground flour	150
	1 tablespoon syrup and 1 pat butter	100
	1 slice Canadian bacon	60
	¾ cup skim milk	90
	TOTAL	500
LUNCH	2–4 tablespoons fiber appetizer*	50
	4 ounces shrimp (steamed)	150
	2 tablespoons cocktail sauce	30
	10 salt-free crackers	100
	2 cups tomato and lettuce salad	50
	1 tablespoon Omega mayonnaise**	100
	¾ cup skim milk	90
	TOTAL	570
MIDAFTERNOON SNACK	¾ cup skim milk or apple juice	90
	1 tablespoon raisins in 4 ounces plain yogurt	80
	TOTAL	170
DINNER	2–4 tablespoons fiber appetizer*	50
	Roman rice and beans**	350
	2 cups lettuce and tomato salad	50
	1 tablespoon Omega mayonnaise**	100
	4″ wedge honeydew melon	100
	TOTAL	650
EVENING SNACK	½ slice stone-ground whole-wheat toast	40
	¾ cup skim milk	90
	TOTAL	130
	GRAND TOTAL	2020

*Recipe for fiber appetizer cocktail appears on page 29.
**Recipe appears in recipe sections following these menus.

SATURDAY

			Calories
BREAKFAST	2–4 tablespoons fiber appetizer*		50
	½ grapefruit		40
	2 eggs any style		200
	1 slice stone-ground whole-wheat bread		75
	¾ cup skim milk		90
	2 teaspoons butter or oil		70
		TOTAL	525
LUNCH	2–4 tablespoons fiber appetizer*		50
	1½ cups macaroni and cheese		340
	1½ cups tomato and lettuce salad		30
	1 tablespoon Omega mayonnaise**		100
	½ cup broccoli		30
	¾ cup skim milk		90
		TOTAL	640
MIDAFTERNOON SNACK	Orange or apple		60
	¾ cup skim milk		90
		TOTAL	150
DINNER	2–4 tablespoons fiber appetizer*		50
	6 ounces turkey (roasted)		300
	½ cup cooked brown rice		70
	Fruit and 1 ounce low-fat cheese		180
		TOTAL	600
EVENING SNACK	1 tablespoon raisins		20
	½ cup yogurt or skim milk		60
		TOTAL	80
		GRAND TOTAL	1995

*Recipe for fiber appetizer cocktail appears on page 29.
**Recipe appears in recipe sections following these menus.

RECIPES FOR
STANDARD OMEGA MENUS

OMEGA MAYONNAISE   *(approximately 2 cups)*

1 egg
1 teaspoon salt
1 teaspoon dry mustard
3 tablespoons lemon juice

½ teaspoon paprika
1¼ cups soy, walnut, wheat germ,
  or linseed oil

1. Put all except oil in blender.
2. Cover blender and run for 10 seconds.
3. Uncover and, while blender is still running, add oil very gradually.
4. Blend until smooth.

NOTE: Reduce amount of oil slightly if mayonnaise is too thick.

OMEGA OIL AND VINEGAR
SALAD DRESSING   *(approximately 2 servings)*

2 tablespoons soy or walnut oil
1 teaspoon red wine vinegar
½ teaspoon dry mustard
½ teaspoon dry oregano leaves
½ teaspoon salt

1 clove garlic, sliced
2 teaspoons chopped shallots or
  onions
2 tablespoons lemon juice.

1. Mix all ingredients in a closed glass jar.
2. Allow to stand for 5–10 minutes.
3. Strain through medium sieve to remove solids.
4. Pour over salad and toss. Adjust to taste with fresh ground pepper.

SHRIMP AND RICE   *(serves 2)*

1½ cups cooked brown rice
2 tablespoons butter
4 tablespoons soy oil

2 large cloves garlic, crushed
¾ pound peeled shrimp
Dash of salt

1. Keep cooked rice hot.
2. Melt butter in frying pan and add oil.
3. Lightly brown garlic in oil and butter.
4. Add shrimp and cook until shrimp are pink.
5. Add salt to taste.
6. Serve over cooked brown rice.

NOTE: Try Basmati rice, a long-grain rice with some of the husk left on.

CREAMED TUNA ON TOAST   *(serves 2)*

1 tablespoon butter
1 tablespoon stone-ground
   whole-wheat flour
¾ cup milk

2½ ounces poached fresh tuna,
   flaked
2 slices stone-ground whole-wheat
   toast
White pepper and salt to taste

1. Melt butter, add flour, and blend to make smooth paste.
2. Add milk gradually. Stir with wire whisk until blended.
3. Cook over low heat until sauce thickens.
4. Add tuna and dash of salt and white pepper to taste.
5. Serve over stone-ground whole-wheat toast.

BROILED FISH   *(serves 1)*

4 ounces fresh bluefish fillet
2 tablespoons lime juice
Dill (optional)

1. Place fish in glass or ceramic bowl.
2. Pour lime juice over bluefish.
3. Let stand 15 minutes at room temperature.
4. Broil in preheated pan for 5–7 minutes or until fish just begins to turn opaque. Do not overcook.
5. Serve at once with additional lime juice. *Optional:* Dot with melted butter.

High-Omega Single-Dish
Traditional Meals

Every culture has its traditional dishes. For example, *pulmetarium,* a one-dish meal of lentils, beans, peas, and chestnut flour or another similar combination was a standard meal of the average working Roman during ancient times. Examples of traditional dishes still enjoyed by the average person are:

- Polenta of middle and southern Europe
- Varnishka of middle European Jews
- Chili, tacos, and enchiladas of Mexico
- Succotash of native Americans

- Rice and fish, tofu, and miso of the Orient
- Hummus of the Middle East

The protein components of dishes mixing legumes and non-legumes are generally in the same proportion: one part legumes (beans, peas, lentils, or peanuts) plus two parts non-legumes (cereals, rice, corn, seeds, and/or nuts). This balance is complementary for essential amino acids. Together the two plant groups provide the right proportions of the ten amino acids that combine to make complete proteins. When vegetables and fruits are added, as well as some fish, dairy food, or meat, traditional one-dish meals prove satisfying and wholesome. To assure acceptance by your family as you switch from their familiar meals, it is best to introduce not more than one new single-dish meal in a week. Repeat the dishes you and your family like, and gradually build a repertoire of favorites.

Special Omegafication tips

There are many ways to "Omegafy" almost any of your favorite dishes. Once you've done that, you can introduce these dishes in your regular Omega diet.

- For breakfast, experiment with fish occasionally. For example, try oyster bisque, Oysters Rockefeller, pickled herring and cream, or the Jewish traditional lox (smoked salmon slices) and whole-grain bagels.
- Use the tasty low-calorie dressings, sauces, desserts, and entrées given in the Easy-thin, Gourmet-thin, and Vegetarian recipes given later in this book. They not only save calories but are great dishes in their own right.
- Many recipes of your own can be "Omegafied" by substituting recommended products from the Omega shopping list for the ones listed in the recipes. For example, use nonhydrogenated soybean, walnut, or wheat germ oil in place of other oils; stone-ground whole-wheat breads and pastas in place of other noodles, pastas or cereals; and replace meat with either fish or fowl.

**Recipes for Nutritionally Complete High-Omega
Single-Dish Meals**

BROILED FALAFEL PATTIES   *(serves 2–4)*

2 cups cooked dry beans
½ cup parsley clusters
3 cloves garlic, pressed
½ teaspoon dry mustard
1 teaspoon cumin
½ teaspoon chili powder

Celery salt to taste
Salt and pepper to taste
1 teaspoon Worcestershire sauce
¼ cup sesame butter (tahini)
1 egg, beaten with 1 tablespoon
    water

1. Puree the cooked beans, parsley, and seasonings in a blender.
2. Combine the remaining ingredients in a large bowl; add the pureed
bean mixture.
3. Drop by spoonfuls (about ten) onto an oiled baking pan. Flatten spoonfuls evenly in pan to make 3″ patties and brush with soy or walnut oil. Bake
15 minutes or broil a few minutes, basting with oil if surface becomes too
crisp.
4. Serve with lettuce and additional tahini in warm pita or separately as
hors d'oeuvres.

CHEESE SOUFFLÉ   *(5 servings)*

4–6 slices stone-ground whole-
    wheat bread
3 cups grated cheese
2 cups milk or ½ cup of milk
    and ½ cup of wine or
    vermouth

3 eggs, beaten
½ teaspoon salt
½ teaspoon Worcestershire sauce
½ teaspoon thyme
½ teaspoon dry mustard
Pepper

1. Layer slices of bread and cheese in an oiled baking dish.
2. Pour milk or milk and wine combination over the cheese and bread.
3. Mix together the eggs and seasonings.
4. Pour egg mixture over the milk-saturated bread and cheese.
5. Allow to stand 30 minutes at room temperature.
6. Place oiled pan in a larger pan of hot water; bake 1 hour in medium
(350° F.) oven until high and brown.
7. Serve immediately.

CURRIED EGGS   *(4–6 servings)*

6–8 large eggs, hard boiled
½ cup shredded Swiss cheese
2 tablespoons butter
3 tablespoons stone-ground
    whole-wheat flour

1 tablespoon curry powder
¼ cup sherry
2 cups milk
Salt and pepper to taste

1. Prepare and have ready the eggs and Swiss cheese.
2. Over low heat, melt butter; gradually stir in flour and curry powder.
3. Add sherry, milk, salt, pepper, and half the cheese gradually while stirring mixture.
4. Slice eggs in half and arrange, yolk up, in oiled baking dish.
5. Spoon curry cheese sauce over eggs and sprinkle with remaining cheese.
6. Serve over 4–6 slices of toast made from stone-ground bread or over 3–4 cups of cooked brown rice.

INDIAN RICE AND BEANS   *(6 servings)*

2 cups cooked kidney beans
5 cups cooked brown rice
2 teaspoons salt
2 cloves garlic, crushed
1 large onion
1–2 medium carrots, chopped
1 stalk celery, chopped
1 green pepper, chopped

⅔ cup chopped parsley
2–3 teaspoons dried basil
1 teaspoon oregano
2 tablespoons soy or walnut oil
2–3 large tomatoes, chopped
Pepper
½ cup grated Parmesan cheese

1. Cook brown rice with salt.
2. Reserve cooked beans and brown rice.
3. Sauté garlic, onion, carrots, celery, pepper, parsley, basil, and oregano together in oil until onions are golden and other vegetables soften.
4. Add cooked beans, tomatoes, and pepper to taste.
5. Combine cooked rice with cheese and fold bean mix into rice mix.
6. Serve hot or at room temperature; garnish with parsley sprigs and an additional sprinkle of cheese.
NOTE: Salad and stone-ground bread are nice accompaniments.

POTATO LATKES   *(2–3 servings)*

½ onion, grated
1 large potato, peeled and
   grated, liquid drained
2 tablespoons whole-wheat
   flour

2 tablespoons parsley
2 eggs, beaten
Salt and pepper to taste
5 tablespoons instant dry milk
Omega oil for frying

1. Combine all ingredients except oil and mix batter well.
2. Form into small pancakes.
3. Heat oil, then fry pancakes in oil.
4. Brown both sides well.
5. Remove from oil when brown; drain on paper towel.
6. Top with applesauce if desired. Serve with a cottage cheese and tomato salad.

FETTUCCINE AL MARCO   *(4 servings)*

½ pound stone-ground whole-   ½ cup chopped parsley
   grain fettuccine or other pasta   2 cups chopped spinach leaves
1½ cups ricotta cheese   Salt and pepper to taste
¼ cup grated Parmesan cheese   Basil
½ cup yogurt   Black olives, sliced
1 egg   Parsley sprigs

1. Cook pasta in rapidly boiling water.
2. Blend cheeses, yogurt, egg, chopped parsley and spinach, and salt and pepper until very smooth.
3. Toss the hot pasta with the sauce.
4. Arrange in bowl or on platter, garnish with basil, sliced olives, and parsley sprigs, and serve immediately.
NOTE: Spinach pasta may be substituted for whole-grain pasta.

GREEK-STYLE SKILLET   *(4 servings)*

1 cup brown rice, raw   ½ teaspoon mint
¼ cup soy granules   ½ teaspoon dill weed
2 tablespoons soy or walnut oil 1 tablespoon parsley flakes
1 medium onion, chopped   Juice of 1 lemon (2 tablespoons)
1 clove garlic, minced   1 cup diced, raw tomato
1 small eggplant, peeled and   1 8-ounce can tomato sauce
   diced
¼ pound green beans, fresh or
   canned

1. Cook brown rice with soy granules.
2. While rice is cooking, sauté onion and garlic in oil until golden.
3. Add eggplant and beans; sauté for 5 minutes more.
4. Add mint, dill, and parsley; sauté another minute while stirring gently to combine ingredients.
5. Add lemon juice, tomatoes, and tomato sauce.
6. Cover and cook for 15 minutes.
7. Place rice and soy mixture in large bowl; serve vegetables over cooked grains.
NOTE: Serve 2 cups yogurt as a side dish. A Greek salad also goes well with this meal.

TOSTADAS   *(6 servings of 2 tostadas each)*

5 cups soft cooked dry beans
1 dozen corn tortillas
4 ripe tomatoes
6 green chilies
1 onion, minced
1 clove garlic, minced
1 teaspoon vinegar
⅛ teaspoon pepper

¼ cup soy or walnut oil
½ pound Monterey Jack or
  cheddar cheese, grated
½ head lettuce, shredded
1–2 fresh tomatoes, chopped
1 onion, finely chopped
1 cup yogurt
1 teaspoon salt

1. Have cooked beans and tortillas ready.
2. Peel and remove seeds of the four ripe tomatoes.
3. Remove seeds from the green chilies.
4. Chop the tomatoes and chilies and mix well with minced onion, garlic, half the salt and pepper, and vinegar.
5. In a dry skillet, heat oil until very hot; add beans.
6. Mash beans with wooden spoon while cooking; sprinkle with remaining salt and pepper.
7. Fry tortillas separately in a small amount of oil, or heat in oven until crisp.
8. Spread beans on tortillas.
9. Top with vegetable sauce.
10. Garnish with cheese, shredded lettuce, chopped tomatoes and onion, and yogurt.

SAVORY RICE   *(4 servings)*

3 cups cooked brown rice
¼ cup dry soybeans, cooked
  with bay leaf (makes ¾ cup)
1–2 tablespoons soy or walnut
  oil
¾ cup chopped onion
2 cloves garlic, crushed

1–2 cups mixed, chopped raw
  vegetables (carrots, celery, 1–2
  mushrooms, sliced bamboo
  shoots, and sprouts)
2 tablespoons soy sauce
Nuts or seeds (e.g., chopped
  walnuts, sunflower seeds)

1. Prepare rice and beans and reserve.
2. Heat oil in heavy skillet.
3. Sauté onion, garlic, and chopped mixed vegetables together until onions are golden and vegetables soften.
4. Stir cooked rice into vegetable mix; add soy sauce.
5. Stir in cooked beans; remove bay leaf.
6. Top with nuts or seeds and serve at once with more soy sauce.

IRISH STEW   *(4–6 servings)*

1½ pounds lean leg of lamb
¾ cups sliced onions
2½ pounds potatoes
Salt and pepper to taste

1 bay leaf
2 cups boiling water or stock
2 tablespoons finely chopped
  parsley

1. Cut lamb into 1½-inch cubes.
2. Peel and slice both onions and potatoes into ⅛″ slices.
3. In bottom of heavy pan, layer potatoes, meat, and onion. Repeat twice, ending with a fourth layer of potatoes on top.
4. Season each layer with salt and pepper.
5. Add the bay leaf.
6. Pour boiling water or stock over the layers.
7. Bring to a boil. Cover tightly. Simmer gently over low heat for about 2½ hours or until done.
8. Shake the pot periodically so that the potatoes do not stick. When done, all the moisture should have been absorbed by the potatoes.
9. Garnish with parsley and serve hot.

WHEAT-SOY VARNISHKES   *(4 servings)*

1 cup dry stone-ground
  macaroni shells, cooked and
  drained
2 tablespoons soy oil or butter
¼–½ pound mushrooms, sliced
1 large onion, chopped
¼ cup blender-cut soybeans

¾ cup bulgur wheat
1 beaten egg
2 cups vegetable or chicken stock
  or water with vegetable
  seasoning added
Salt and pepper
Parsley sprigs

1. Cook and drain pasta.
2. Sauté mushrooms and onion in oil or butter; remove from skillet; set aside in another dish.
3. Turn off heat.
4. In same skillet, mix beans, wheat, and egg until grain is coated.
5. Stir-fry coated grain over medium heat until dry.
6. Pour vegetable or chicken stock over grain, cover tightly, lower heat, and cook 10 minutes.
7. When grains are fluffy, toss with onion and mushrooms. Add cooked macaroni and remaining oil or butter.
8. Salt and pepper to taste; garnish with parsley sprigs.
9. Serve warm or at room temperature as main dish or side dish.

18

Lose Weight and Keep It Off: The Three-Phase Omega Weight-Loss Program

Provided you do not have irreversible obesity from permanently damaged weight-control physiology, you can expect this slow but sound method to get your weight down and keep it down with minor effort. You will be able to suppress the weight yo-yoing so common with other diets.

The Omega Weight-Loss Program consists of three phases:

Phase I: The dietary normalizing phase

Start the program by going on the Everyday Standard Omega Diet for four to six months. Your regimen should include the fiber "appetizer" but can be carried out with or without the Mega-Omega Supplement Program. This phase is designed to normalize your calorie-handling physiology for what comes later. You may lose all the weight you need at this stage, even without paying much attention to calorie intake.

Phase II: The physical normalizing phase

In this phase you will add a regular aerobic exercise program to your diet. Almost everyone should exercise, even if only to initiate a program of brisk walking daily. Exercise is especially important for those with a weight problem. It further normalizes the body's calorie-handling physiology. In this phase, you may lose enough weight without concentrating on calorie intake.

Phase III: The weight-normalizing phase

This is a specific weight-loss phase using the low-calorie Omega weight-loss diets, which are offered in three options:

1. Omega Easy-thin
2. Omega Gourmet-thin
3. Omega Veggie-thin

These options can be used either by following the menus or in a free choice form.

OBESITY—A SIGN OF MODERN MALNUTRITION

Many health problems arise primarily from malnutrition; ironically, obesity is one of them. Conventional weight-loss programs focus on the symptoms—the excess weight itself—rather than on the underlying disease process causing the obesity—the malnutrition. The most popular therapeutic weight-loss programs only monitor weight. They do not take health and physiology into account. None are nutritionally complete, therapeutic programs specifically designed to correct the underlying malnutritional cause of obesity. As a result, these other programs induce harmful weight fluctuations—the yo-yo syndrome—in about 80 percent of the cases. Drastic weight fluctuations of more than 10 percent of body weight in a short period of time may cause health-damaging deposits of arterial plaques and other problems that are more debilitating and unhealthy than just staying overweight.

If you are about 20 percent over your ideal body weight, you should follow all of the suggested guidelines below. These are based on the body weight of a 150-pound person. Adjust them to your own needs by adding or subtracting proportionally.

When body weight is 20 percent or more above the healthful normal level, the condition is described as obesity. Nutritionists, physicians, scientists, and everyone interested in good health have declared obesity an enemy, and perhaps a killer. Compared with persons of normal weight, the obese tend to have:

- High blood pressure
- Elevated levels of cholesterol in the blood
- Non–insulin-dependent diabetes
- Cancers (colon, rectum, and prostate in men; gallbladder, breast, uterus, ovaries, and cervix in women)

To assume that obesity itself is the cause of illness and that its removal is the cure misses the point: Obesity is just one more symptom of a disorder caused by the synergistic modern malnutrition—part of the modernization disease syndrome—which adversely affects the appetite-controlling appestat in the brain as well as the heat-controlling, calorie-burning thermogenic system.

Obesity isn't just too much body fat—it indicates complex damage to the body chemistry.

Obesity, stress, and your genetic makeup

Once obesity becomes a problem, it compounds other stresses and reveals other genetic weaknesses. The high circulating levels of insulin and fats that often develop in obese individuals can contribute to cardiovascular, blood sugar, and other disorders and thus lead to other problems.

We all know people who don't seem to eat much—they may even eat substantially less than those around them—but are nevertheless fat. The latest research has confirmed that there really are many people who eat little and still gain weight. The weight they develop is called "no fault fat," and it results not because the basal metabolism is too low, but because transient thermogenesis, the operation of the heat-making system within the body, does not respond correctly to drafts and brief cooling with extra heat production around the core organs. This is why many overweight people are very sensitive to cold.

"Brown fat"—different from other fat

A special kind of fatty tissue called brown fat is responsible for heat production. Different from the usual body fat, which is yellow or white, brown fat is found packed around the abdominal organs and along the spine and at the back of the neck. Each brown fat cell is packed with energy factories—mitochondria. Although most of our cells have these mitochondria, brown fat cells contain them in large numbers. It is the special job of mitochondria to create heat. The rich blood supply in brown fat tissue then rapidly removes the heat to other parts of the body and keeps them warm.

A normal body with brown fat in good working order uses a high percentage of the daily intake of calories just to keep itself warm. After all, the internal temperature is usually 98.6 degrees Fahrenheit, usually appreciably warmer than the air around the body. (Movement also creates some heat, which makes you warmer when you exercise.) As with other aspects of cold adaptation, the Omega-3 fatty acids are directly involved in the mechanisms that turn brown fat into body heat.

Researchers have become very interested in brown fat. They've found a connection between inadequate thermogenesis (heat generation) by brown fat and the accumulation of weight even on low-calorie diets.

Inadequate heat-producing brown fat can be a difficult problem. Those lucky people with a healthy thermogenic mechanism simply burn off the calories from their occasional hot fudge sundae, but without competent brown fat that doesn't happen. Weight is added. There is evidence that as the obese reduce calorie intake their bodies actually fight the loss of weight by burning off even fewer calories.

Putting brown fat to work

In laboratory tests, the natural steroid dehydroepiandrosterone (DHEA) increases the ability of mice to consume food without gaining weight, apparently by activating the brown fat system. In humans, the ability to make DHEA decreases as one grows older, which may account in part for added weight and heightened cold sensitivity with age.

Special amino acids are now being used experimentally in weight-loss programs because they are part of the chemical chain that stimulates brown fat to produce heat. Omega-3 EFA are also a part of that chain.

Omega-3 EFA regulate brown fat

The Omega-3 EFA regulate brown fat, the depositing of regular fat, and hair growth and in this way affect cold-sensitivity and calorie burning in response to cold. (They also regulate skin tanning.) In my study, a number of the forty-four subjects noticed that they lost their lifelong cold-sensitivity after taking linseed oil supplements for some months. Additionally, the Omega-3 EFA appeared to improve skin texture, color, and ability to tan. Above all, overweight subjects stopped years of weight yo-yoing and found it much easier to achieve and maintain normal weight.

In polar climates, fish and marine mammals—seals, whales, and polar bears—are protected by a fat layer that contains abundant super-polyunsaturated Omega-3 DHA and EPA. It also contains plentiful cholesterol. However, native Eskimos who exist on this diet have healthy hearts and arteries just the same. Rich amounts of DHA and EPA in their food protect their cardiovascular system from harm.

Using aerobic exercise to escape diet plateaus

Most dieters become frustrated by a slowing in weight loss at some time during their dieting. This slowing down occurs because the body's metabolism goes into a plateau to protect itself. The human body is very frugal, squeezing every possible calorie out of the food consumed. It slows down its use of calories when presented by what the body perceives as a potentially dangerous starvation situation—i.e., a reduced intake of calories. Aerobic exercise can be used to force your frugal body to use more calories and in that way jog you off the plateau.

Aerobic exercise forces your metabolism out of its self-induced slump and speeds up the burning of fat as fuel. Exercise may even activate the body's heat makers—brown fat cells.

Why some foods make you hungry

In overweight people, the natural appetite mechanism is also abnormal, being easily provoked by simple carbohydrates such as sugar. To compound the problem, high-sugar foods are usually stripped of the nutrients the body needs to metabolize the sugars they contain.

Without natural fiber to slow the digestion and absorption of sugars, they enter the bloodstream very quickly. This provokes an insulin surge from the pancreas, freeing the glucose in the blood to be rapidly absorbed by the cells of the body—including adipose cells—which quickly convert the glucose to fat. The liver also turns glucose into fat and sends the fat on to the adipose tissues for storage.

The insulin effect is so intense that about an hour later, the blood glucose falls to such a low point that you're hungry again and forced to eat more and more to satisfy an inner need, resulting in a binge. We don't understand all the reasons, but many people experience this hunger response to foods largely made up of sugar and white flour. Once they start eating these foods they are in trouble.

Sugar addiction—a serious problem

The concept of "allergy addiction" offered by some physicians may also explain part of this phenomenon. When someone has become sensitive to a substance because of overexposure, the body goes through a process of accommodation. Eventually the uncomfortable allergic symptoms are quieted only by the provocative substance itself. This leads to an addictive pattern similar to alcoholism. Soon after the substance is taken, a strong desire for it returns—just to avoid withdrawal symptoms. With sugary, highly refined foods, the repetition of this cycle thousands of times creates overweight. It also damages both physiology and psychology, thus creating the addictive personality.

When an Omega-3 EFA deficiency or an Omega-3/Omega-6 imbalance and distorted dietary cofactors are present—as they often are—health problems, including obesity, are multiplied. If you suffer from sugar-addiction weight gain, ordinary weight-loss diets lead to additional stress, which compounds the problems, leading to the very real dangers of cyclical weight gain and loss (the yo-yo syndrome).

PHASE I: THE STANDARD OMEGA DIET
FOR FOUR MONTHS

Your first step here is to go on Phase I, the Everyday Standard Omega Diet, for four months (see chapter 17). This is a program, not a diet, and it necessary—or even beneficial—to count calories. However, this program must be followed for a minimum of four months. Many of my study subjects followed it for six months and lost weight permanently during that time. (You may need to try the Omega Supplement Program at the same time.)

The Ten Nonbreakable Weight-Loss Rules

Here are ten easy-to-follow rules for the program. You must follow them exactly for the program to work at its best. Do not make any substitutions and do your best to hold on to your willpower through your first few weeks on the program.

1. Take three teaspoons of linseed oil daily. Each teaspoon should be taken directly before meals. It can be taken in juice or followed by juice.

2. Use no oils other than linseed, walnut, soy, or wheat germ oil in cooking or as food oils. Check labels; be sure the mayonnaise or salad oils you use are made only from these oils.

3. Use no margarine or solid shortening. For toast or cooking, use only butter or Omega oils. (Limit butter to one teaspoon daily.)

4. Take a premeal fiber-yogurt cocktail before at least two of every three of your daily meals. (See page 29 for a recipe for the fiber cocktail and directions for taking it.)

5. Take a one-a-day vitamin-mineral supplement. If you feel the need for additional supplementation, add:

- 500 milligrams of vitamin C
- 50–100 IU of vitamin E
- 25 micrograms of selenium
- 50 micrograms of chromium from yeast. (This essential trace element, low in many diets, is required for insulin to do its job in regulating blood sugar.)

6. Use only bread, pasta, or pastries made either entirely from stone-ground whole-wheat flour or from a mixture of whole wheat, soy, or other whole grains. All cereals—oats, rice, bulgur wheat, buckwheat, millet, corn, or other grain—should be unrefined and whole grain.

7. Eat a minimum of two whole fruits daily; do not drink fruit juices but use pureed drinks. The exception is a small glass of juice, which can be taken with the linseed oil supplement.

8. Eat a minimum of two servings of fatty fish—salmon, mackerel, herring, or trout—each week. The fats in these fish are unlike those in meat. (If fresh fish is not available, use frozen fish or well-drained canned

fish.) Keep red meat down to two or three meals per week, and even then substitute chicken whenever possible.

9. Eat three meals daily. Do not skip meals. Each meal should include foods from each of the basic three food groups identified in chapter 15. Or just follow the Standard Omega Diet menus in chapter 17).

10. Although you don't need to count calories, at this point there are some food restrictions in this program:

- No sugar
- No soft drinks, except low-calorie drinks
- No cakes, cookies, bread, pasta, ice cream, or candies that are made using either sugar or white flour (the only exception is your birthday or wedding cake)
- No snack foods such as corn chips and potato chips
- No fried foods
- Use fructose for a sweetener, but sparingly. Frozen fruit concentrate can be used as sweetener for beverages or desserts.
- Eat only small quantities of nuts or seeds (one small handful a day). The nuts must be fresh or roasted, not fried.

The Omega Weight-Loss Program will be easier to follow if your menus include soup, a raw salad, a plate or side dish of beans or brown rice, and plentiful vegetables cooked *al dente*. For snacks, try raw carrots, celery, cauliflower—or drink a glass of water.

Follow each meal with a small fruit such as an apple and about an ounce of soft or medium-hard cheese. This sort of meal will take time to eat. Slow eating is required on the diet. If you take the fiber cocktail with water ten or fifteen minutes before meals, your full stomach will affect the satiety centers in the brain. Use the Omega snacks listed later.

PHASE II: THE AEROBIC EXERCISE PROGRAM

The people who say "Use it or lose it" are right: Disuse is your body's enemy as much as misuse. A sedentary life-style weakens all your systems and accelerates the aging process. Some insurance companies reduce life insurance premiums for people who do aerobic exercise for thirty minutes three times a week because exercise:

- Slows the aging process
- Alleviates tension
- Reduces weight
- Lowers serum fat
- Lowers blood pressure
- Dissipates anxiety
- Suppresses appetite

If you don't feel your present health is optimum, or are over age forty, consult your physician before you begin any exercise program.

After you have normalized your food intake via the Standard Omega Diet for four to six months, and assuming that you are in reasonable health, you must begin a regular aerobic exercise program. There is evidence that simply reducing calories without adequate exercise causes overweight individuals to use less calories, as though the body's thermogenic mechanisms were out to save every last calorie you eat.

Heart rate measurement

The definition of aerobic exercise is exercise that gets the heart rate up to 180 beats a minute minus your age, for more than ten minutes. This produces what is called a "cardiopulmonary training effect" for each minute it is sustained in excess of ten minutes. For example, for aerobic benefits:

- If you are twenty, your aerobic heart rate level is 180 minus $20 = 160$.
- If you are forty, your aerobic heart rate level is 180 minus $40 = 140$.
- If you are sixty, your aerobic heart rate level is 180 minus $60 = 120$.

To measure your heart rate, lightly hold your index and third fingers on a pulse point at the side of the neck or on your wrist and count beats for ten seconds. Then multiply the result by six. However, maintaining simple breathlessness over which you can speak is a simple guide to determining that you are in an aerobic condition.

The program basics

As mentioned, aerobic exercise produces the so-called cardiopulmonary training effect, with improved heart and body circulation. Never mind counting your pulse, just sustain mild continuous breathlessness. Every minute of continuous breathlessness in excess of ten minutes brings on the "training effect," building coronary artery and general circulation.

In a sensible aerobic exercise program, mild breathlessness should be sustained for more than ten minutes, ideally worked up to at least twenty to thirty minutes every other day. At the very least, over a period of some weeks you should work up to the point where you can walk vigorously up to thirty minutes to an hour.

After a few weeks, your physical condition permitting, you can try getting up on your toes for a few jogging or dance steps and then walk again, in this way gradually working your way up to alternately walking and jogging or even full jogging for thirty minutes. Swimming, dancing, skipping rope, cycling, tennis volleying, Frisbee throwing, and boomerang throwing are all good aerobic exercises, provided you keep the mild breathlessness going in excess of ten minutes.

Following this simple regimen alone can lower high blood fats in many people, as can EFA, fiber, and B-vitamin supplements. Taken together, these steps will put most people back on the road to health.

A Walking and Jogging Program

For many people, jogging or a combination of walking and jogging is the exercise of choice. It can be done anywhere with a minimum of equipment. (However, a good pair of running shoes is a worthwhile investment.) Jogging is not just running.

The Jogging Program

Before you begin: Evaluate your general health status; consult your physician for special health problems.

Before each run: Do six stretching and six strengthening exercises. (Do thirty seconds of each of the stretchers and ten each of the strengtheners.)

Your first goal: briskly walking two miles in thirty minutes without getting winded

Use the joggers' "six sixes":

1. Six stretching exercises
2. Six strengthening exercises
3. Six minutes of warm-up jogging followed by
4. Increased exertion to six times six (thirty-six) breaths per minute, done easily, without becoming winded, aiming for the aerobic threshold, ten to fifteen minutes
5. Increase activity slightly each week until you are able to jog six miles in sixty minutes or three miles in thirty minutes.
6. Do the six stretchers to cool off.

THE SIX STRETCHERS

The six stretching exercises that follow should start your aerobic program every time. They take only ten minutes and provide the framework for all athletics. If you are stretching correctly, it should not hurt, nor should your muscles feel stiff or sore afterward. After the stretching, warmup exercises are necessary. The best kind of warm up is to walk or jog slowly for about half a mile and then gradually increase your pace.

Almost everyone should be able to do one set of each of these six stretching exercises. Stretch slowly, holding the stretch for thirty seconds. Then progress to three sets of slow continuous stretching. Stretching too fast or too far will cause microscopic tears that shorten the muscle, the exact opposite of what you want to achieve. Work from the feet up.

1. Achilles tendon and gastrocnemius stretch

- Lean forward with your hands against a wall.
- Move your feet away from the wall, keeping heels on the ground and knees straight, until you sense a gentle pull on the calves.
- Hold for thirty seconds.
- Repeat two or three times.
- Keeping heels on the ground, flex the knees to stretch the Achilles tendons at the back of the ankles.

2. Hamstring and lumbar stretch

- Slowly bend down to touch your toes with your fingertips.
- Take fifteen to thirty seconds to slowly stretch as far down as you can. It may take several months before you can actually touch your toes. *Do not pump up and down.*
- Hold position for thirty seconds.
- Repeat two or three times.

3. Reverse lumbar stretch

- Tilt pelvis forward, and stretch the small of the back.
- Follow by tilting pelvis backward, and again stretch the small of the back, this time in the reverse direction.
- Hold each motion for thirty seconds.
- Repeat two or three times.

4. Trochanter stretch

- Move the hips to one side.
- Hold for thirty seconds.
- Now slowly bend the torso away from the hips to stretch the lateral trochanter tendons, which run over the outer thigh below the hips.
- Hold for thirty seconds.
- Stretch the other side in the same manner.
- Repeat two or three times for each side stretch.

5. Groin stretch

- Spread the legs into a partial split.
- Place hands on ground to control balance and amount of stretch.
- Hold each stretch for thirty seconds.
- Repeat two or three times.

6. Shoulder stretch

- Swing arms in a complete vertical circle.
- Place hands on back and shoulders, stretching the arms.
- Keep rotating arms for thirty seconds.

NOTE: Arthritic pains or pains in the bursa indicate a need for Omega-3 oil and cofactoring vitamins, minerals, and fiber. If you have difficulty with any of these stretching exercises, try performing them after a hot shower or hot bath. The degree of muscular elasticity will be greatly increased. Do *not* try these exercises while standing on a wet, slippery surface.

THE SIX STRENGTHENERS

Everyone should be able to do ten repeats of the following six strengtheners. Work up to three sets of ten each, holding for ten seconds in the appropriate isometric cases. (It may take several months to work slowly up to the recommended levels.)

1. Shin and foot strengtheners

- Sit on a high chair or bench with your legs dangling above the floor.
- Place an appropriate five-pound weight (available from sporting goods stores or call a local health club for a source) on the toes and lift the foot slowly upward.
- Hold the foot at knee level for ten seconds.
- Repeat ten times, repeat in two or three sets of ten.

2. Kneecap straightener

- Sit on a high chair or bench with legs dangling above the floor.
- Attach a five-pound weight to the ankle.
- Lift the leg out straight and hold at full extension for ten seconds.
- Repeat ten times; then do two or three more sets of ten.
- Try to increase weight on each ankle every two weeks. (Do not exceed fifty pounds.)

3. Quad strengthener

* Do ten shallow knee bends. You can perform them as step-ups or double steps if you prefer.
* Repeat ten times; repeat in two or three sets of ten.

4. Stomach muscle strengthener

* Lie on back with hands behind head, keeping upper back and head elevated.
* Raise left knee and touch with opposite elbow.
* Return leg and arm to original position, then repeat with right knee and opposite elbow.
* Alternate in pedaling motion, extending legs without touching floor.
* Start with three sets of ten.
* Try to build up to twenty to thirty cycles per set, then repeat that three times for a total of sixty to ninety cycles.

5. Low back strengthener

* Lying on your stomach, do full back arches, lifting chest, arms, and legs off the floor.
* Lift and hold for ten seconds.
* Repeat. Try to build up to three sets of ten for a total of thirty.

6. Arm and chest strengthener (knee push-up)

* Lie on floor, face down, legs together, with knees bent and feet on floor.
* With hands palms down on the floor under your shoulders, push your upper body up off floor until your arms are fully extended and your body is in a straight line from head to knees.
* Repeat. Try to build up to three sets of ten.

For the Vigorous—Test Yourself

One day a week, after the six-minute warmup and after jogging for your regular time and distance, stretch your muscles, then find the limit of your wind by doing interval training: Run short, fast runs of 100, 200, 400, and 800 yards and one mile. (Walk between runs to get your breath.)

On the other days of the week, pace yourself, going slowly, to see how long you can run to test your strength and endurance limits.

PHASE III: THE OMEGA WEIGHT-LOSS DIET

Many people will find Phase I or Phase I and Phase II sufficient to bring their weight under satisfactory and permanent control. Others, however, need a further program to lower their weight.

For that, use the 1,200-calorie Omega Easy-thin, Gourmet-thin, or Veggie-thin Weight-Loss Diet for two to four weeks, then resume the Standard Omega Diet for two weeks. Continue alternating two to four weeks on one of the Omega weight-loss diets followed with two weeks on the Standard Omega Diet until your ideal weight has been achieved. You should be able to achieve your target weight in six months or less.

Find your best weight

Try to find a reasonable weight: Use the chart indicating ideal weights developed by the Association of Life Insurance Medical Directors in 1983. It shows ideal weight per age and body build to be much higher than in a previous chart issued about twenty-five years ago. Follow the new weights.

Use the charts below to find your target weight and your calorie intake. After you know your target weight, subtract that from your present weight and roughly calculate the number of dieting days you'll need to achieve your weight goal. People use calories at different rates because of differences in their metabolism, so you may lose weight somewhat faster or slower than average.

Weigh yourself, without clothes, twice a week when you get up in the morning. Enter your weight on a photocopy of the "Chart of Your Weight Loss" chart. On the average, a safe and sensible weight loss for a person of about 150 pounds is approximately one-quarter pound per day, or one to two pounds each week. You are trying to get this weight off permanently; don't rush it.

Expect a temporary plateau

Do not be misled by rapid weight loss during the first week; this is the result of water loss, not fat or tissue loss. The water will be replaced if you go off the diet. After the initial water loss, you may find yourself at a discouraging weight plateau for many days or weeks. Don't get discouraged. During that time other physiological adjustments are occurring. Keep to your diet during this plateau, and don't forget your exercise program—it is vital for achieving further weight loss. After a time you will break through the plateau level. If you continue your diet, you will reach your target weight.

Your Ideal Weight

For ages 25–59
Subtract 5 pounds for men, 3 for women if you weigh yourself nude.

| | MEN | | | WOMEN | | |
Height	Small frame	Medium frame	Large frame	Small frame	Medium frame	Large frame
4'10"				102–111	109–121	118–131
4'11"				103–113	111–123	120–134
5'0"				104–115	113–126	122–137
5'1"				106–118	115–129	125–140
5'2"		131–141	138–150	108–121	118–132	128–143
5'3"		133–143	140–153	111–124	121–135	131–147
5'4"		135–145	142–156	114–127	124–138	134–151
5'5"		137–148	144–160	117–130	127–141	137–155
5'6"	136–142	139–151	146–164	120–133	130–144	140–159
5'7"	138–145	142–154	149–168	123–136	133–147	143–163
5'8"	140–148	145–157	152–172	126–139	136–150	146–167
5'9"	142–151	148–160	155–176	129–142	139–153	149–170
5'10"	144–154	151–163	158–180	132–145	142–156	152–173
5'11"	146–157	154–166	161–184	135–148	145–159	155–176
6'0"	149–160	157–170	164–188	138–151	148–162	158–179
6'1"	152–164	160–174	168–192			
6'2"	155–168	164–178	172–197			
6'3"	158–172	167–182	176–202			
6'4"	162–176	171–187	181–207			

Copyright © Metropolitan Life Insurance Co., 1983

How long should you diet?

Never continue any weight-loss diet phase for more than two to four weeks. After a maximum of four weeks dieting, resume the Standard Omega Diet for two weeks. If further weight loss is desired, then return to one of the Omega-thin Diets. Continue alternating two to four weeks on and two weeks off until you achieve your desired weight. Or choose a two-week reducing diet phase alternated with two weeks on the Standard Omega Diet. If you suffer any side effects such as weakness or dizziness, go off the reducing diet at once and start again later at a slightly higher calorie level.

Worried about regaining the loss you do achieve? Set a trigger weight of three to four pounds over your target weight. If you find your weight creeping above this, return to one of the Omega diets for three to seven days of dieting.

Calories Needed to Maintain Weight with Light Activity

(Reduce by 5–10% for each decade over 25 years)

Your wt. in lbs.	Calories (men)	Calories (women)	Your wt. in lbs.	Calories (men)	Calories (women)
100	2500	2000	160	3500	2800
110	2700	2100	170	3600	2900
120	2800	2300	180	3800	3000
130	3000	2400	190	3900	3100
140	3100	2600	200	4100	3200
150	3300	2700	210	4300	3300

Time Needed to Lose a Given Number of Pounds on a Given Calorie Intake

(Add 33% to allow for a 2-week "holiday" every four weeks. Add 100% to allow for a 2-week "holiday" every two weeks.)

If you need this many calories to maintain wt:	Then it will take this many diet days to lose:			
	5 lbs.	10 lbs.	20 lbs.	40 lbs.
On a 1200-calorie diet				
1800	30	60	120	240
2000	22	45	90	180
2200	18	35	70	140
On a 1400-calorie diet				
1900	35	70	140	280
2100	25	50	100	200
2300	20	40	80	160
On an 1800-calorie diet				
2400	30	60	120	240
2600	22	45	90	180
2800	18	35	70	140

Chart Your Weight Loss

Starting weight	Weeks on which you are on the program. (Count the "holiday" weeks as well as diet weeks.)											
	1	2	3	4	5	6	7	8	9	10	11	12
190												
185												
180												
175												
170												
165												
160												
155												
150												
145												
140												
135												
130												
125												
120												
115												
110												
105												
100												

Circle the number that indicates your target weight. Make an X each week in the box that corresponds to your actual weight and the week of the program. Connect the X's with a line to show your progress in reaching your target weight.

Before you start

Before starting any of the Omega diets, review the general Omega program guidelines:

- Do your food shopping according to the Omega Shopping guide (see chapter 16). Select only foods that are on the list.
- Get ready for the Omega Weight-Loss Diet by completing the Standard Omega Diet for four months and following the exercise program for two months.
- Finally, commit yourself totally to the Omega Weight-Loss Diet in advance.

During Phase III you have these options:

1. You can stay on the already familiar Standard Omega Diet of Phase I, using the Omega Shopping Guide as before, and merely reduce all portions by one-half. The Standard Omega Diet is based on about 2,500 calories; half the amount of food will provide between 1,200 and 1,300 calories daily.

2. You can go on one of the three appetite-suppressing high-protein Omega Weight-Loss diets that follow in this book.

Twenty tips for making dieting easier

Many of these have already been stated. Nevertheless, they are repeated here because they are so important for achieving weight loss.

1. Avoid refined flour, breads, and pastas; use stone-ground flour, breads, and pastas.

2. Avoid use of any hydrogenated oil or southern oils and margarine.

3. Strictly limit bread and butter.

4. Keep alcoholic beverages to a minimum.

5. Use decaffeinated coffee and tea (water-decaffeinated rather than chemically decaffeinated) and use a little fructose or a nonsugar sweetener if necessary in place of sugar. If you don't like black coffee use a little skim milk instead of cream or artificial creamer.

6. Use low-calorie lemon, vinegar, vinaigrette, or mustard sauces for salad dressings (see recipes).

7. Use lemon juice and spices on vegetables instead of butter. (Refer to the Gourmet-thin Diet suggestions for additional ideas.)

8. Use only lean meat, low-fat cottage cheese, and protein-fortified skim milk (less than 1 percent fat). (All meat portions in the menus provided represent cooked and drained meats without skin, fat, or bones.)

9. Avoid luncheon meats, sausages, or hot dogs, which are all very high in saturated fat.

10. Use no cooking oils except as noted in the recipes. Use nonstick Teflon or Silverstone pans to reduce need for cooking oils.

11. Eat slowly. Enjoy animated and interesting conversation. Allow satiety to build up. Stop when full. Never stuff yourself, and always be prepared to leave food on your plate.

12. Confine snacks to celery, carrots, cucumber slices, pickles, or other suggested snacks from the list on page 176. Snack as often as you wish. Drink a glass of water when hungry. (NOTE: Smokers and ex-smokers should eat one medium-sized carrot daily.)

13. Do not skip meals or snacks. It will only make you ravenous later and can cause you to go off the diet.

14. When away from home, use commercial high-fiber biscuits or crackers at each meal, according to directions, as substitutes for fiber cocktail.

15. If you are allergic to any food, make sensible substitutions. (See chapter 21.)

16. Avoid all ice cream, pastries, pies, cookies, candy, pasta, or other products made with white flour and refined sugar. Avoid canned fruits in heavy sugar syrup.

17. Increase physical activity. It is almost as important as the Omega therapeutic weight-loss diets. To lose a pound of body weight you must burn off 3,500 calories in excess of the calories consumed.

18. As part of general health care, some people find that trying a specific program of relaxation (see references in Appendix B) can help with a variety of problems, including compulsive eating.

19. Never try to lose weight when pregnant.

20. Each day of the diet take one RDA-complete multivitamin and multimineral supplement and your premeal fiber cocktails with a glass of water.

The three 1,200-calorie Omega diets you can choose from

Don't worry, you will not get bored on the diet. You can select from any of the three Omega weight-loss diets, or combine them. All of them provide the Omega-3 nutritional missing link and exclude antinutrients.

- The *Omega Easy-thin Diet* is attractive because of the simplicity of food preparation.
- The *Omega Gourmet-thin Diet* may be right for you if you are willing to spend time and effort in food preparation.
- The *Omega Veggie-thin Diet* is for those who insist on a vegetarian menu.

All these Omega weight-loss diets are restricted to about 1,200 calories daily. Since they are "Omegafied" versions of medically approved diets *(Merck Manual)*, they are also all nutritionally complete. All three diets are:

Low-fat	High-EFA
Low-isomer	High-antioxidant
Low-sugar	Protein-balanced
Low-cholesterol	Appetite-suppressing

The Veggie-thin Omega Diet—pros and cons

The Veggie-thin Omega Diet is a low-protein diet and is therefore less appetite-suppressing and tissue-protecting than the Omega Easy-thin Diet or the Omega Gourmet-thin Diet. To make a vegetarian version of either the Easy-thin or Gourmet-thin Omega diets, simply substitute some of the nutritionally complete traditional single-dish meals for the fish, chicken, or meat dishes on the menu. However, the total protein intake may be too low for the stresses of weight reduction and for adequate hunger supression. If that is true for you, select one of the other diets.

How to choose and use one of the Omega diets

Free-choice Omega diet. You can select foods or meal menus from the lists in this book and consume them in moderate amounts until your hunger is satisfied. This will provide you sufficient protein and fiber and keep sugar low to help suppress your appetite.

No-choice Omega diet. For better appetite and weight control follow the diet regimens as given, because these provide calorie and portion control. Each day's menu provides the RDA of both polyunsaturated EFA families (6 to 8 percent of calories as Omega-6 and 1 to 2 percent as Omega-3) and is low in saturated fat. All the Omega diets exclude antinutrients and provide about 1,200 calories per day in three meals and two snacks. Your daily intake following these systems will be 40 percent protein, 35 percent carbohydrate (plus dietary fiber), and 20 to 25 percent fat.

No matter which diet or which eating plan you select, never reduce calories by more than one-half your normal intake and never go below 1,200 calories daily for a 150-pound person—reducing calories any further makes it difficult to get a nutritionally balanced diet. Also, very rapid weight loss can cause dangerous electrolyte deficiencies, which can precipitate heart attacks, congestive heart failure, and other problems.

The Omega Weight-Loss Program is designed not just to take pounds off but to keep them off. It goes beyond current reducing diets, which induce weight fluctuations in about 80 percent of the people who use them. Be patient; correcting the causes of overweight takes time. What you want is to eliminate the causes of your weight problems, and not just settle for quick weight loss that will be reversed later.

How to Omegafy any diet you prefer

Most commercial diets can be "Omegafied," or nutritionally normalized. The weight-loss diets in this chapter are "Omegafied" versions of standard, medically approved, high-protein–high-fiber diets. The high protein in weight-loss programs adds two great advantages: strong appetite suppression (to reduce calorie intake) and a sparing action on tissue protein to ensure the weight loss is fat. You can also substitute one commercial high-protein liquid meal (e.g., Cambridge Diet, University Diet) per day, provided it has been Omegafied.

To Omegafy a liquid protein meal, add one-half teaspoon (20 calories) of nonhydrogenated cold-pressed soy, walnut, or wheat germ oil or a quarter teaspoon linseed oil. Take your premeal fiber cocktail before drinking the liquid protein, and follow the fiber cocktail with a glass of water. In addition, be sure to take a complete multivitamin/mineral supplement tablet daily. *Never substitute more than one protein drink meal a day for normal foods.*

Omega Snacks

Post this list somewhere in your kitchen—your refrigerator door might be an excellent spot. The list will help remind you of the large number of good foods that are also good for you.

Carob powder for "chocolate" skim milk	Low-salt bouillon
Carrot sticks	Omega nuts—walnuts, chestnuts, hazel nuts, beechnuts
Cauliflower or broccoli flowerets	Potato chips cooked in Omega oils
Celery stalks	Potato salad
Fresh fruits	Sliced lox (Nova is best)
Graham crackers	Smoked oysters, mackerel, or herring
Granola bar	Toasted pieces of stone-ground whole-wheat bread
High-fiber cereals	Tomato juice
Lettuce leaves	Tuna fish salad on stone-ground whole-wheat crackers
Lettuce and tomato salad	Zucchini sticks
Low-calorie yogurt	
Low-fat cottage cheese	
Low-fat milk	

THE EASY-THIN OMEGA DIET MENUS

The Easy-thin Omega Diet is a simple day-by-day menu program emphasizing foods that require a minimum of preparation effort. Because nutritional balance has been built into each day's meals, it is best to follow the menu plan as closely as possible. If you do make substitutions, keep within the general diet guidelines previously given, and make substitutions as close as possible in calorie and nutrient balance.

SUNDAY

		Calories
BREAKFAST	2–4 tablespoons fiber appetizer*	50
	½ grapefruit	40
	½ cup low-fat cottage cheese	95
	1 slice stone-ground whole-wheat toast	75
	½ cup skim milk	60
	TOTAL	320
LUNCH	2–4 tablespoons fiber appetizer*	50
	7 ounces shrimp, steamed	180
	1 slice stone-ground whole-wheat bread	75
	1½ cups tomato and lettuce salad with lemon juice	35
	½ cup skim milk	60
	TOTAL	400
MIDAFTERNOON SNACK	1 small apple	40
	½ cup skim milk or ½ cup plain yogurt	60
	TOTAL	100
DINNER	2–4 tablespoons fiber appetizer*	50
	8 ounces chicken (broiled)	200
	1 cup green beans	30
	1½ cups green salad with mild vinegar	35
	2″ melon wedge	25
	TOTAL	340
EVENING SNACK	1½ cup skim milk or low-fat cottage cheese	60
	2–4 stalks celery or carrot sticks	10
	TOTAL	70
	GRAND TOTAL	1230

*See recipe on page 29 for fiber appetizer cocktail.

MONDAY

		Calories
BREAKFAST	2–4 tablespoons fiber appetizer*	50
	½ orange	40
	1½ ounces ham (baked or broiled)	155
	1 slice stone-ground whole-wheat bread	75
	½ cup skim milk	60
	TOTAL	380
LUNCH	2–4 tablespoons fiber appetizer*	50
	2 cups vegetable-soy salad	90
	2 teaspoons low-calorie dressing	90
	½ cup skim milk	60
	TOTAL	290
MIDAFTERNOON SNACK	½ ounce Gouda cheese	50
	1 cup bouillon	10
	TOTAL	60
DINNER	2–4 tablespoons fiber appetizer*	50
	8 ounces bluefish (broiled)	270
	1 cup broccoli (steamed)	40
	½ cup skim milk	60
	TOTAL	420
EVENING SNACK	½ cup skim milk or yogurt	60
	Celery and carrots	10
	TOTAL	70
	GRAND TOTAL	1220

*See recipe on page 29 for fiber appetizer cocktail.

TUESDAY

		Calories
BREAKFAST	2–4 tablespoons fiber appetizer*	50
	½ grapefruit	40
	½ cup Bran Flakes or Shredded Wheat	75
	½ cup skim milk	60
	1 ounce baked ham	105
	TOTAL	330
LUNCH	2–4 tablespoons fiber appetizer*	50
	2 ounces roast beef	150
	1 ounce Swiss cheese	110
	1½ cups tomato and lettuce salad	30
	½ cup skim milk	60
	TOTAL	400
MIDAFTERNOON SNACK	½ cup skim milk	60
	TOTAL	60
DINNER	2–4 tablespoons fiber appetizer*	50
	8 ounces Cornish hen or chicken (broiled or roasted)	200
	1 cup green beans (steamed)	30
	1 cup cauliflower (raw or steamed)	30
	2" wedge melon	30
	TOTAL	340
EVENING SNACK	¼ cup cottage cheese	55
	2–4 stalks celery or leafy vegetable	15
	TOTAL	70
	GRAND TOTAL	1200

*See recipe on page 21 for fiber appetizer cocktail.

WEDNESDAY

		Calories
BREAKFAST	2–4 tablespoons fiber appetizer*	50
	½ orange	40
	¾ cup low-fat cottage cheese on	135
	1 slice stone-ground whole-wheat bread	75
	TOTAL	300
LUNCH	2–4 tablespoons fiber appetizer*	50
	¾ cup tuna (water-packed) on	190
	1½ cups tomato and lettuce salad	30
	½ slice stone-ground whole-wheat bread	40
	TOTAL	310
MIDAFTERNOON SNACK	½ cup skim milk	60
	TOTAL	60
DINNER	2–4 tablespoons fiber appetizer*	50
	4 ounces lean roast beef	300
	½ cup broccoli (steamed)	20
	½ slice stone-ground whole-wheat bread	40
	½ cup unsweetened applesauce	50
	TOTAL	460
EVENING SNACK	2 stalks celery or leafy vegetable	10
	½ cup skim milk	60
	TOTAL	70
	GRAND TOTAL	1200

*See recipe on page 29 for fiber appetizer cocktail.

THURSDAY

		Calories
BREAKFAST	2–4 tablespoons fiber appetizer*	50
	½ grapefruit	40
	1 large egg (poached or boiled)	90
	1 ounce baked ham	100
	½ slice stone-ground whole-wheat bread	40
	TOTAL	320
LUNCH	2–4 tablespoons fiber appetizer*	50
	¾ cup low-fat cottage cheese, tossed with	145
	1½ cups tomato, mushrooms, lettuce	75
	½ cup skim milk	60
	TOTAL	330
MIDAFTERNOON SNACK	1 cup bouillon	10
	1 stalk celery or 1 small carrot	10
	TOTAL	20
DINNER	2–4 tablespoons fiber appetizer*	50
	8 ounces salmon with lemon	265
	1 cup brussels sprouts (steamed)	30
	½ cup berries or ½ large apple	35
	1 cup skim milk	90
	TOTAL	470
EVENING SNACK	2 stalks celery	10
	½ cup plain yogurt or skim milk	60
	TOTAL	70
	GRAND TOTAL	1210

*See recipe on page 29 for fiber appetizer cocktail.

FRIDAY

		Calories
BREAKFAST	2–4 tablespoons fiber appetizer*	50
	2–3 dried prunes (or 1/2 citrus)	50
	1/2 cup low-fat cottage cheese on	95
	1 slice stone-ground whole-wheat bread	75
	1/2 cup skim milk	60
	TOTAL	330
LUNCH	2–4 tablespoons fiber appetizer*	50
	8 ounces chicken (broiled)	200
	1-1/2 cups lettuce and tomato salad with mild vinegar	30
	1/2 cup skim milk	60
	TOTAL	340
MIDAFTERNOON SNACK	4 ounces tomato juice	25
	1 tablespoon raisins in 1/2 cup plain yogurt	85
	TOTAL	110
DINNER	2–4 tablespoons fiber appetizer*	50
	5 ounces lean lamb roast	265
	1-1/2 cups spinach and tomato salad with lemon juice	35
	TOTAL	350
EVENING SNACK	3–4 stalks celery or 1 carrot	20
	1/2 cup skim milk	60
	TOTAL	80
	GRAND TOTAL	1210

*See recipe on page 29 for fiber appetizer cocktail.

SATURDAY

		Calories
BREAKFAST	2–4 tablespoons fiber appetizer*	50
	1/2 grapefruit	40
	3/4 cup 40% Bran or Shredded Wheat with	100
	3/4 cup skim milk	90
	TOTAL	280
LUNCH	2–4 tablespoons fiber appetizer*	50
	3/4 cup tuna (water-packed)	190
	1-1/2 cups lettuce and tomato salad with lemon	40
	TOTAL	280
MIDAFTERNOON SNACK	1/2 orange or 1 small (1/2 cup) apple	40
	1/2 cup skim milk	60
	TOTAL	100
DINNER	2–4 tablespoons fiber appetizer*	50
	5 ounces lean roast pork	340
	1 cup cauliflower (steamed)	30
	1 cup spinach salad with lemon juice	40
	TOTAL	460
EVENING SNACK	4 lettuce leaves	10
	1/2 cup yogurt or skim milk	60
	TOTAL	70
	GRAND TOTAL	1190

*See recipe on page 29 for fiber appetizer cocktail.

19

The Gourmet-thin Omega Diet and Recipes

The Gourmet-thin Omega Diet is a high-protein and high-fiber, Omega-balanced weight-loss diet. The "gourmet" dishes featured either cost more or require greater preparation than those in the other diets.

As with the Easy-thin Diet, you can follow a *free-choice* regimen, adhering to the weight-loss rules given below, or follow the *no-choice* Gourmet-thin menus at the end of this chapter.

Suggested Dishes for
Free-Choice Diet Regimen

Breakfast

- Eat fruit or mixed fruits as often as possible—pineapple, papaya, mango, melons, peaches, or berries. Temperate fruits are best.
- Try lox (sliced smoked salmon) or other breakfast fish dishes such as oysters and herring.
- Use decaffeinated coffee and tea.

Lunch or Dinner

- Devil, curry, or barbecue shrimp, crab, or lobster (use lemon and garlic sauce).
- Use Chinese stir-fried dishes and vegetable quiches.
- Prepare any of these as featured dishes:

Fresh fruit salads	Stews
Eggplant dishes	Pepper steak
Grilled cheese and ham sandwiches	Chicken liver pâté
	Chicken cacciatore
Lamb cooked with herbs and spices or mustard sauces	Marinated meats
	Broiled tomatoes

- For dessert, have a baked apple or stewed or broiled fresh fruits.

Weight-loss rules

These rules are given elsewhere in this book; they are provided here as a reminder and review.

1. You should be shopping the Omega way, have been on the Standard Omega Diet for four to six months, and be exercising regularly before going on this weight-loss diet.
2. Reduce calories, but no more than half your usual intake and to no less than 1,200 calories per day under any circumstances.
3. Note your target weight and how long it will take you to get there, including diet holidays (see pages 170–172).
4. Do not be misled by rapid initial weight loss or discouraging plateaus.
5. Avoid sweets, ice cream, candy, cookies, sugary canned fruits, white bread and butter, and pastas and pastries made with refined white flour. Also avoid margarine and hydrogenated or southern oils. Use nonhydrogenated walnut, linseed, soybean, or wheat germ oil and stone-ground flours, breads, and pastas and low-fat protein-fortified milk, cottage cheese, and yogurt. When traveling, use a fiber powder, wafer, or tablet such as Metamucil, Fiber Med, or Fiber Full as a substitute for the fiber cocktail (fiber appetizer).
6. Restrict alcohol; drink decaffeinated coffee or tea and try it black (with fructose or a sugar substitute if needed).
7. Use lemon juice on vegetables and lemon juice or low-calorie dressings on salads.
8. Use lean meats with fat removed; avoid cold cuts, sausages, or hot dogs.
9. In place of hydrogenated cooking oils, use Teflon or Silverstone no-stick pans.
10. Eat slowly; stop before you are full; never eat until you feel stuffed; leave food on your plate rather than overeat.
11. Snack any time on carrots, celery, or lettuce, or drink a glass of water.
12. Do not skip meals.
13. Exercise regularly.
14. Do not try to lose weight if you are pregnant, unless you first consult your physician.
15. Take a holiday from weight-loss dieting every two to four weeks.

GOURMET-THIN OMEGA MENU

SUNDAY

			Calories
BREAKFAST	2–4 tablespoons fiber appetizer*		50
	½ cup fresh fruit		50
	½ cup Bran Flakes		60
	½ cup skim milk		60
		TOTAL	220
LUNCH	2–4 tablespoons fiber appetizer*		50
	Tuna cheese grill**		200
	½ cup creamy coleslaw**		35
	½ cup berries		45
		TOTAL	330
MIDAFTERNOON SNACK	1 small apple		40
	½ cup skim milk or ½ cup plain yogurt		60
		TOTAL	100
DINNER	2–4 tablespoons fiber appetizer*		50
	Veal cutlet Romano**		300
	½ cup broccoli		20
	1½ cup salad with low-calorie French dressing**		75
	2″ melon wedge		25
		TOTAL	470
EVENING SNACK	½ cup skim milk, cottage cheese, or cottage cheese mousse**	TOTAL	60
		GRAND TOTAL	1180

*See recipe on page 29 for fiber appetizer cocktail.
**See recipe section following these menus.

MONDAY

			Calories
BREAKFAST	2–4 tablespoons fiber appetizer*		50
	½ cup fresh fruit		50
	Cottage Cheese Grill Maxine**		260
		TOTAL	360
LUNCH	2–4 tablespoons fiber appetizer		50
	Chicken salad		210
	2 slices stone-ground whole-wheat Melba toast		60
		TOTAL	320
MIDAFTERNOON SNACK	½ ounce Gouda cheese		50
	1 cup bouillon		10
		TOTAL	60
DINNER	2–4 tablespoons fiber appetizer*		50
	Indian curry**		245
	½ cup rice		90
	½ cup green beans		15
		TOTAL	400
EVENING SNACK	½ cup skim milk or yogurt		60
	Celery stalk or carrot		10
		TOTAL	70
		GRAND TOTAL	1210

*See recipe on page 29 for fiber appetizer cocktail.
**See recipe section following these menus.

TUESDAY

		Calories
BREAKFAST	2–4 tablespoons fiber appetizer*	50
	½ cup gourmet fruit	50
	1 egg (boiled or poached)	90
	1 slice stone-ground whole-wheat toast with curry powder	70
	½ cup skim milk	60
	TOTAL	320
LUNCH	2–4 tablespoons fiber appetizer*	50
	Tuna Salad Roget**	165
	1 slice stone-ground whole-wheat toast	45
	½ cup skim milk	60
	TOTAL	320
MIDAFTERNOON SNACK	½ small apple	40
	½ cup skim milk or plain yogurt	60
	TOTAL	100
DINNNER	2–4 tablespoons fiber appetizer*	50
	5 ounces filet mignon with mushrooms**	250
	½ baked potato	45
	1½ cups salad with 2 tablespoons low-calorie Roquefort dressing**	60
	2″ melon wedge	25
	TOTAL	430
EVENING SNACK	½ cup skim milk or cottage cheese	60
	2–4 stalks celery or carrots	20
	TOTAL	80
	GRAND TOTAL	1250

*See recipe on page 29 for fiber appetizer cocktail.
**See recipe section following these menus.

WEDNESDAY

			Calories
BREAKFAST	2–4 tablespoons fiber appetizer*		50
	½ cup gourmet fruit		50
	1½ slices stone-ground whole-wheat French toast**		230
		TOTAL	330
LUNCH	2–4 tablespoons fiber appetizer*		50
	1 cup Zesty Onion Soup**		80
	Baked macaroni and cheese**		100
	½ cup skim milk		60
		TOTAL	290
MIDAFTERNOON SNACK	½ cup skim milk		60
	½ small apple		40
		TOTAL	100
DINNER	2–4 tablespoons fiber appetizer*		50
	Broiled Scallops Reverend Jacques**		120
	½ cup asparagus (steamed)		15
	½ slice stone-ground whole-wheat bread		35
	½ cup skim milk		60
		TOTAL	280
EVENING SNACK	1 ounce cheddar cheese		110
	½ cup skim milk		60
		TOTAL	170
		GRAND TOTAL	1170

*See recipe on page 29 for fiber appetizer cocktail.
**See recipe section following these menus.

THURSDAY

			Calories
BREAKFAST	2–4 tablespoons fiber appetizer*		50
	½ cup gourmet fruit		50
	1 cup oatmeal		130
	½ cup skim milk		60
		TOTAL	290
LUNCH	2–4 tablespoons fiber appetizer*		50
	Spinach Salad Deluxe** with		210
	2 tablespoons red wine dressing**		50
	1 slice stone-ground whole-wheat Melba toast		30
		TOTAL	340
MIDAFTERNOON SNACK	1/2 cup plain yogurt		60
		TOTAL	60
DINNER	2–4 tablespoons fiber appetizer*		50
	4 ounces quick-poached salmon** with		250
	2 tablespoons melted butter and lemon		90
	1/2 cup broccoli		20
	2″ melon wedge		30
		TOTAL	440
EVENING SNACK	½ cup skim milk or cottage cheese		60
	2–4 stalks celery or small carrots		20
		TOTAL	80
		GRAND TOTAL	1210

*See recipe on page 29 for fiber appetizer cocktail.
**See recipe section following these menus.

FRIDAY

		Calories
BREAKFAST	2–4 tablespoons fiber appetizer*	50
	½ cup gourmet fruit	50
	1 poached egg on stone-ground whole-wheat toast	160
	TOTAL	260
LUNCH	2–4 tablespoons fiber appetizer*	50
	Cold salmon platter**	280
	2 tablespoons low-calorie mayonnaise**	30
	TOTAL	360
MIDAFTERNOON SNACK	½ cup skim milk	60
	TOTAL	60
DINNER	2–4 tablespoons fiber appetizer*	50
	Lamb kebab**	200
	½ cup rice	90
	1 cup green beans (steamed)	40
	½ cup skim milk	60
	TOTAL	440
EVENING SNACK	½ cup skim milk or yogurt	60
	2–4 stalks celery or small carrots	20
	TOTAL	80
	GRAND TOTAL	1200

*See recipe on page 29 for fiber appetizer cocktail.
**See recipe section following these menus.

SATURDAY

			Calories
BREAKFAST	2–4 tablespoons fiber appetizer*		50
	Omega omelette**		200
	1 slice stone-ground whole-wheat bread		70
	½ cup skim milk		60
		TOTAL	380
LUNCH	2–4 tablespoons fiber appetizer*		50
	Tuna tacos**		360
	1 cup bouillon		10
		TOTAL	420
MIDAFTERNOON SNACK	½ orange or 1 small apple		40
		TOTAL	40
DINNER	2–4 tablespoons fiber appetizer*		50
	Peppercorn steak**		160
	8 fresh or frozen asparagus tips		20
	Salad with low-calorie French dressing**		80
		TOTAL	310
EVENING SNACK	Lettuce, celery, and carrots		20
	½ cup plain yogurt or skim milk		60
		TOTAL	80
		GRAND TOTAL	1230

*See recipe on page 29 for fiber appetizer cocktail.
**See recipe section following these menus.

GOURMET-THIN OMEGA DIET RECIPES

Main Dishes

BAKED MACARONI AND CHEESE
(4 servings, 100 calories each)

1 cup elbow macaroni, cooked
1 egg, beaten
⅓ teaspoon salt
1 teaspoon garlic salt
2 teaspoons dried parsley

8-ounce can tomato sauce
2 tablespoons minced onion
Pinch cayenne pepper
2 tablespoons grated extra sharp
  cheddar

1. Cook macaroni according to package directions.
2. Combine cooked macaroni with other ingredients in a one-quart casserole.
3. Bake in preheated 350-degree oven for 45 minutes.

BROILED SCALLOPS REVEREND JACQUES
(2 servings, 125 calories each)

½ pound bay scallops
1 tablespoon soy oil (or 2 pats
  butter)

1 tablespoon sherry
½ teaspoon paprika
Salt and pepper to taste

1. Place scallops in a shallow nonstick baking dish.
2. Spread oil or dot butter evenly over scallops.
3. Sprinkle with sherry, some paprika, salt, and pepper.
4. Broil for 2 minutes under highest flame.
5. Turn scallops.
6. Sprinkle with additional paprika.
7. Broil for an additional 5 minutes until browned and moisture has evaporated.

COLD SALMON PLATTER
(1 serving, 285 calories)

3 ounces cold poached salmon
Crisp lettuce leaves
1 tomato, cut in wedges

1 tablespoon low-calorie Omega
  mayonnaise (see page 200)
Lemon juice and capers
1 Melba toast rectangle

1. Arrange salmon on a bed of lettuce.
2. Garnish with tomato wedges, mayonnaise, and Melba toast.

COTTAGE CHEESE GRILL MAXINE

(1 serving, 270 calories)

⅓ cup low-fat cottage cheese
2 teaspoons fructose
¼ teaspoon cinnamon

1 tablespoon chopped walnuts
1 slice stone-ground whole-wheat toast

1. Combine first four ingredients and spread on the toast.
2. Broil for 5 minutes at 400 degrees (keep approximately 4 inches from heat source).

FILET MIGNON AND MUSHROOMS

(4 servings, 250 calories each)

4 5-ounce tenderloin steaks trimmed of fat

½ cup dry white or red wine
½ pound fresh mushrooms, sliced

1. Put steaks and ¼ cup of wine in a nonstick skillet.
2. Heat over high flame until wine evaporates and the steaks begin to brown.
3. Turn steaks and add mushrooms.
4. Cook another 4–5 minutes to taste (until mushrooms are slightly browned).
5. Remove steaks to heated platter and add remaining wine to skillet.
6. Cook and stir until wine boils, then pour over steaks and serve at once.

INDIAN CURRY

(2 servings, 245 calories per serving)

1 tablespoon oil or butter
2 heaping tablespoons chopped onion
1 clove garlic, finely minced
1 tablespoon curry powder (approximate)
½ pound fresh tomatoes or 1 tablespoon tomato paste, thinned with water

½ pound lean, fresh leg of lamb, shrimp, or poultry, cubed into bite-sized pieces
Salt
Lemon juice or vinegar

1. Put oil or butter, onions, and garlic in a nonstick skillet and cover.
2. Cook over low heat for 4–5 minutes, but do not allow onions to brown.
3. Add curry powder; mix well and cook for another 4–5 minutes on low heat, stirring continually.
4. Add the tomatoes and meat, mix well and cover. (See note below if using shrimp.)

5. Cook slowly for as long as possible, until almost dry.

6. Add water to form a thickish sauce and continue to cook slowly, until the meat is tender. Add salt to taste and lemon juice or a teaspoon of vinegar to taste.

7. Serve over ½ cup cooked brown rice.

NOTE: For fish, shrimp, precooked meat, or vegetables, prepare the curry sauce first, then add the main ingredients and heat to warm.

LAMB KEBABS

(6 servings, 200 calories each)

1½ pounds boneless leg of lamb, trimmed of fat and cut into 1" cubes
6 tablespoons lemon juice
¼ teaspoon dried thyme or rosemary

1½ teaspoons garlic salt
1 tablespoon Worcestershire sauce
2 green peppers, cut in chunks
4 tomatoes, cut in wedges
6 small onions, cut in chunks

1. Put lamb cubes in dish with lemon juice, and add thyme or rosemary, garlic salt, and Worcestershire sauce.

2. Add just enough water to cover lamb and marinate 2 hours at room temperature, or 8–10 hours in the refrigerator.

3. Drain meat, saving marinade, and, alternating pieces of lamb with chunks of pepper, tomato, and onion, thread meat on six skewers.

4. Broil 15–20 minutes over hot coals or in the broiler, turning frequently and brushing with marinade.

OMEGA OMELET

(1 serving, 200 calories)

1 egg
Salt to taste
¼ teaspoon soy or walnut oil

1 slice stone-ground whole-wheat bread

1. Lightly fork-whip egg and salt to taste.

2. Heat oil in nonstick skillet until very hot.

3. Add beaten egg; slowly count to ten so egg begins to set.

4. Shake skillet lightly and, when egg is almost firm but still slightly liquid, use fork to loosen one end of omelet and roll it over on itself.

5. Slide omelet onto plate, letting egg heat finish the cooking. Serve with one slice bread.

VARIATIONS: Sprinkle chopped vegetables on the egg mixture while it is still cooking, or top with tomato sauce, soy sauce, or crushed fresh berries.

PEPPERCORN STEAK

(4 servings,
160 calories each)

2 tablespoons whole
   peppercorns
4 lean 4-ounce steaks
Soy or walnut oil

Worcestershire sauce, Tabasco
   sauce, or lemon juice to taste
Fresh parsley or watercress

1. Use mortar and pestle to coarsely crack the peppercorns, or pound with hammer.
2. Press cracked peppercorns into both sides of steaks and refrigerate for 1 hour.
3. Wipe a nonstick skillet with soy or walnut oil.
4. Brown steaks quickly on both sides to taste, then remove to a serving dish.
5. Sprinkle lightly with Worcestershire and Tabasco or lemon juice. Garnish with parsley or watercress.

QUICK-POACHED SALMON

(2 servings,
150 calories each)

2 4-ounce salmon steaks

1 tablespoon low-calorie
   mayonnaise or 1 teaspoon
   melted butter or lemon juice to
   taste

1. Boil enough salt water to cover fish.
2. Lower heat to simmer and add steaks.
3. Simmer 7–10 minutes until fish just turns opaque. *Do not cover.*
4. Remove fish from water; remove skin and bone.
5. Serve with warmed low-calorie mayonnaise or 1 teaspoon melted butter or lemon juice.

STIR-FRIED TURKEY TENDERLOINS

(4 servings,
245 calories each)

1 tablespoon soy or walnut oil
1 pound turkey white meat,
   cooked, cut into 1″ cubes
1 onion, peeled, halved, and
   thinly sliced
1 cup fresh mushrooms, sliced
1 8-ounce can water chestnuts,
   drained and sliced

1 cup diagonally sliced celery
   pieces
¾ cup turkey or chicken broth,
   skimmed of fat
1 green bell pepper, seeded and
   diced
Soy sauce to taste

1. Heat a very small amount of oil in a large nonstick skillet or electric frying pan.
2. Add turkey cubes and stir-fry for 2 minutes.
3. Add onion and mushrooms and stir-fry for 1 minute.
4. Add remaining ingredients, lower heat.
5. Simmer, uncovered.
6. Stir frequently for about 10 minutes, until broth evaporates.

SHRIMP CREOLE

(4 servings, 220 calories each;
90 calories for rice)

½ cup brown rice, cooked
2 tablespoons soy or walnut oil
½ cup diced onion
1 garlic clove, minced
1 medium green bell pepper, seeded
1 cup sliced mushrooms
½ cup chopped celery
1 cup canned tomatoes, drained and chopped (reserve liquid)

¾ cup bottled clam juice
1 bay leaf
Dash pepper
1½ pounds shrimp, shelled and deveined
1 tablespoon chopped fresh parsley

1. Cook rice according to directions. Follow remaining steps as rice cooks.
2. Heat oil in two-quart saucepan.
3. Add onion and garlic; sauté in oil until onion is softened.
4. Add green pepper, mushrooms, and celery and sauté 5 more minutes.
5. Add tomatoes, reserved liquid, clam juice, bay leaf, and pepper.
6. Cover and simmer for 20 minutes, stirring occasionally.
7. Stir in shrimp and continue simmering 3–5 minutes, until shrimp turn pink.
8. Remove bay leaf and serve garnished with parsley over cooked rice.

TUNA CHEESE GRILL

(1 serving,
250 calories)

1 slice of stone-ground whole-wheat toast or small stone-ground whole-wheat pita
1 teaspoon butter (optional)
¼ medium tomato, sliced
1½ ounces canned, flaked, water-packed tuna, drained

1 teaspoon Omega mayonnaise (see page 200)
½ teaspoon Dijon mustard
⅛ teaspoon salt
Dash pepper
1 ounce low-fat American cheese

1. Butter one side of toast and place, buttered side down, on baking sheet or foil. (If pita is used, open the pocket fully.)
2. Arrange tomato slices on toast or in pita pocket and set aside.
3. In a small bowl, combine remaining ingredients except cheese.
4. Spoon mixture over tomato slices and top with cheese.
5. Broil 3–5 minutes, 3 inches from heat source, or until cheese melts and is lightly browned.

TUNA TACOS

(2 servings,
360 calories each)

2 teaspoons soy or walnut oil
½ cup sliced onions
2 garlic cloves, minced
½ cup chopped tomato
½ cup tomato sauce
Pinch of minced oregano leaves
Salt and pepper to taste

Hot sauce to taste
4 ounces canned, water-packed, flaked tuna, drained
2 6″ tortillas (wheat or corn)
2 ounces cheddar cheese, shredded
½ cup shredded lettuce

1. Heat oil and sauté onion and garlic in a 9-inch nonstick skillet for 5 minutes, until onion slices are translucent.
2. Add tomatoes, tomato sauce, pinch of oregano, salt, pepper, and hot sauce.
3. Cook, stirring occasionally, for 5 minutes. Stir in tuna and cook until heated through.
4. Bake tortillas on baking sheet at 300 degrees for 5 minutes.
5. Remove from oven and immediately fold each tortilla to form a pocket.
6. Fill each pocket with half the tuna mixture.
7. Top with cheese and lettuce shreds.

TURKEY TIDBITS

*(4 servings,
175 calories each)*

½ pound fresh mushrooms,
  sliced
1 large onion, peeled, halved,
  and thinly sliced
½ cup dry sherry

1½ cups fat-skimmed turkey or
  chicken broth (homemade or
  canned)
1 pound turkey tenderloin,
  cooked, cut into 1″ cubes

1. Combine all ingredients in a large nonstick skillet.
2. Cover and simmer 5–6 minutes, stirring frequently until onions are slightly crisp.
3. Uncover. Continue stirring until nearly all the liquid has evaporated (3–4 minutes).

VEAL CUTLET ROMANO

*(4 servings,
300 calories each)*

2 egg whites
2 tablespoons soy or walnut oil
6 tablespoons stone-ground
  wheat flour, sifted
1 pound veal cutlets, cut thin
  and pounded.

Paprika
Salt and fresh ground pepper
8-ounce can tomato sauce
¼ cup grated extra sharp
  Romano cheese

1. Fork-whip egg whites and oil together in shallow bowl.
2. Put flour in another shallow bowl.
3. Dip veal pieces first in flour, then in egg mixture, then in flour again.
4. Arrange on nonstick cookie sheet and bake in very hot oven (450 degrees).
5. Turn with spatula and sprinkle with paprika, salt, and pepper. Bake an additional three to four minutes more.
6. Arrange cutlets in shallow heat-proof serving dish; pour tomato sauce over veal and top with grated cheese.
7. Return to oven for 3–4 minutes, until cheese is melted and bubbly.

ZESTY QUICK ONION SOUP

*(2 servings,
80 calories each)*

8 ounces commercially
  prepared onion soup, fat
  removed and ready to eat

2 Melba toast rounds
2 teaspoons freshly grated
  Romano cheese

1. Heat soup according to instructions on the can.
2. Ladle into individual ovenproof bowls, float toast rounds on soup, and sprinkle with cheese.
3. Place soup bowl under preheated broiler and broil until cheese melts and turns golden brown.

Gourmet-thin Omega Salad Dressings

FRENCH DRESSING
*(4 servings,
30 calories each)*

1 tablespoon soy or walnut oil
5 tablespoons chicken stock
1 clove garlic, peeled
½ teaspoon minced fresh (or ¼
   teaspoon dried) tarragon

½ teaspoon minced fresh parsley
2 leaves fresh basil, minced
1 tablespoon sherry vinegar
1 tablespoon lemon juice
Salt and fresh ground pepper

1. Combine oil, stock, garlic, and herbs in a small bowl and let them marinate for 2 hours.
2. Add the vinegar, lemon juice, salt, and pepper and mix well with a fork.
3. Store covered in a refrigerator; use within a week.

OMEGA MAYONNAISE
(1 cup, 18 calories per tablespoon)

2 eggs
Salt to taste
1 teaspoon paprika
½ teaspoon mustard

¼ cup skim milk
Juice of one lemon
1 tablespoon soy or walnut oil

1. Beat eggs, salt, paprika, and mustard together.
2. Gradually beat in the milk and lemon juice.
3. Stir over a very low flame or in top of double broiler until thick; beat in oil.
4. Refrigerate several hours before using.

MUSTARD SALAD DRESSING
*(3 tablespoons,
35 calories per tablespoon)*

2 tablespoons lemon juice
2 teaspoons Omega oil
Pinch of fructose

¼ teaspoon paprika
⅛ teaspoon salt
⅛ teaspoon dry mustard

1. Combine all ingredients in a covered pint jar.
2. Shake well.
3. Store in refrigerator.

RED WINE DRESSING
*(1 cup,
25 calories per tablespoon)*

3 tablespoons soy oil
¼ cup water
Pinch of cayenne pepper

3 tablespoons red or white wine
   vinegar
½ cup dry red wine
Pinch of fructose

1. Combine all ingredients in a covered pint jar.
2. Shake well.
3. Store in refrigerator.
VARIATIONS: Add 5 tablespoons crumbled blue cheese, 2 teaspoons dry mustard, or 1 beaten raw egg.

ROQUEFORT DRESSING

*(1½ cups,
15 calories per tablespoon)*

1 cup plain yogurt
¼ teaspoon ground pepper
1 teaspoon salt

2 teaspoons vinegar
2 ounces Roquefort cheese
Garlic salt to taste

1. Combine all ingredients in the blender at high speed until smooth.
2. Store in refrigerator.

Salads

CHICKEN SALAD

*(6 servings,
210 calories each)*

3 cups bite-sized pieces
  chicken meat
1 cup finely minced celery
1 medium onion, finely minced
¼ cup chopped dill pickle
1 tablespoon low-calorie
  Omega mayonnaise (see
  page 200)

¼ cup mock sour cream (page
  206)
1 tablespoon lemon juice
Paprika
Salt and pepper to taste
Crisp lettuce leaves

1. Toss together chicken, celery, onion, and pickle.
2. Combine mayonnaise, sour cream, and lemon juice and fold into salad.
3. Toss lightly and sprinkle with paprika, salt, and pepper to taste.
4. Chill before serving on bed of crisp lettuce.

CREAMY COLESLAW

*(6 servings,
30 calories each)*

1 tablespoon skim milk
1 teaspoon horseradish
1 carrot, grated
1 teaspoon garlic powder

¼ teaspoon pepper
⅓ cup plain low-fat yogurt
½ teaspoon salt
2 cups shredded cabbage

1. Thoroughly combine all ingredients except cabbage.
2. Toss cabbage with mixed dressing ingredients until smoothly and evenly coated.
3. Refrigerate in sealed container until served.

SPINACH SALAD

(1 serving, 215 calories)

2 cups raw spinach leaves, washed
4 raw mushrooms, sliced
1 scallion, sliced
Garlic salt to taste
1 ounce low-fat cheese, diced

½ ounce boiled ham, diced
Pepper to taste
Any low-calorie Omega dressing (see preceding recipe section)
1 tomato, cut into wedges

1. Combine all ingredients except tomato and dressing.
2. Toss, add dressing, and toss again before serving.
3. Arrange on salad plate; place tomato wedges on top of salad.

TUNA SALAD WITH FRUIT

(1 serving, 180 calories)

1 cup shredded iceberg lettuce
2 tablespoons chopped green onions
¼ cup sliced celery

½ cup tuna, water-packed
½ large pink grapefruit, sectioned
½ cup sliced tomato

1. Toss lettuce, onion, and celery.
2. Arrange on plate. Put tuna in the center and surround with fruit sections and tomato slices.
3. Serve with low-calorie Omega dressing (see preceding recipe section)
VARIATION: Try substituting chicken for tuna.

TUNA SALAD ROGET

(1 serving, 160 calories)

¼ cup finely chopped celery
½ cup finely chopped carrots
2 teaspoons lemon juice
2 teaspoons low-calorie Omega mayonnaise (see page 200)
½ teaspoon minced onion
½ teaspoon brown mustard

¼ teaspoon salt
Dash of pepper
3 ounces canned, flaked, water-packed tuna, drained
2 iceberg or romaine lettuce leaves

1. Combine all ingredients except tuna and lettuce and let stand at room temperature for 15 minutes.
2. Add tuna and mix well (if too dry, add 1–2 tablespoons water).
3. Serve tuna on lettuce leaves.

Low-Calorie Gourmet Sauces

BASIC LOW-CALORIE
BROWN SAUCE

*(24 tablespoons,
15 calories per tablespoon)*

2 tablespoons butter or soy or walnut oil

2 tablespoons stone-ground whole-wheat flour

¼ cup diced carrots

¼ cup diced celery

¼ cup diced onions

¼ cup tomato puree

2 cups water

2 packets instant beef broth

2 bay leaves

1 garlic clove, minced

⅛ teaspoon ground pepper

Pinch of dried thyme

1. Heat butter or oil in medium saucepan over medium heat until bubbly.
2. Add flour and cook, stirring constantly, for 3 minutes.
3. Add carrots, celery, and onion and continue to stir until vegetables are lightly browned (about 5 minutes).
4. Remove from heat and stir in remaining ingredients.
5. Return to stove, heat to bring mixture to a boil, then reduce heat and simmer for 45 minutes. Stir occasionally.
6. Allow to cool slightly, remove bay leaves.
7. Transfer to blender and process sauce until smooth.
8. Serve over beef, lamb, rice, noodles, or bread.

BASIC LOW-CALORIE
WHITE SAUCE

*(36 tablespoons,
15 calories per tablespoon)*

2 tablespoons butter or soy or walnut oil

2 heaping tablespoons stone-ground whole-wheat flour

2 cups hot skim milk

⅛ teaspoon salt

Dash white pepper

Dash ground nutmeg (optional)

1. Heat butter or oil in small saucepan until bubbly.
2. Add flour and cook over low heat, stirring constantly, for 3 minutes.
3. Remove from heat and, using wire whisk, gradually stir in heated skim milk.
4. Stir until smooth.
5. Add salt, pepper, and nutmeg.
6. Return to stove and cook over medium heat, stirring continually until sauce thickens.
7. Reduce heat as low as possible; cook, stirring occasionally, for an additional 15 minutes.
8. Serve over poultry and seafood.

LOW-CALORIE CHEESE SAUCE

*(4½-cup servings,
150 calories each)*

2 tablespoons butter or soy or walnut oil
2 tablespoons flour
1 cup skim milk

2 ounces Gruyère or hard cheese, shredded
¼ teaspoon salt
Dash of white and dash of red ground pepper

1. Heat butter or oil in small saucepan over medium heat until bubbly.
2. Add flour and cook, stirring continually for 2 minutes.
3. Set aside.
4. In second small saucepan, heat milk to boiling, then remove from heat.
5. Add flour mixture to the milk a little at a time, beating well with a wire whisk until milk and flour are blended.
6. Cook over medium heat, stirring until thickened.
7. Add cheese, salt, and pepper and continue to stir until all the cheese is melted.
8. Reduce heat as low as possible; cook for 30 minutes, stirring occasionally.
9. Serve over cooked cauliflower, broccoli, asparagus, or potatoes. Top the cooked vegetable with sauce, then broil until lightly browned.

LOW-CALORIE CURRY SAUCE

*(4½-cup servings,
90 calories each)*

1⅓ tablespoons butter or soy or walnut oil
2 tablespoons minced onion
2 tablespoons stone-ground whole-wheat flour

1 to 2 teaspoons curry powder
1½ cups skim milk, heated
½ teaspoon salt
Dash white pepper

1. Heat butter or oil in small saucepan until bubbly.
2. Add onion and sauté until softened.
3. Add flour and cook over low heat, stirring continually, for 3 minutes.
4. Add curry powder; continue stirring for 1 minute.
5. Remove from heat. Using wire whisk, gradually stir in heated milk for 1 minute; add salt and pepper.
6. Cook over low heat, stirring frequently, for an additional 10 minutes.
7. Serve hot over eggs, noodles, seafood, or chicken.

LOW-CALORIE FRENCH WINE AND CHEESE SAUCE

(40 tablespoons, 12 calories each)

2 cups skim milk
Pinch cayenne pepper
½ teaspoon salt
Pinch freshly grated nutmeg
½ teaspoon dry mustard

4 teaspoons arrowroot or 2 tablespoons cornstarch
¼ cup sherry or dry vermouth
⅓ cup (3 ounces) Swiss or Gruyère cheese, grated

1. Put milk, cayenne, salt, nutmeg, and mustard in nonstick saucepan and bring to a rapid boil over high heat.
2. Combine the arrowroot and wine in a small bowl and add to the sauce.
3. Stir over low flame until slightly thickened.
4. Remove from heat and stir in cheese.
5. Stir before serving hot over broccoli, green beans, asparagus, chicken, or white fish.

Spreads, Syrups, and Dips

DIET BUTTER

(50 calories per tablespoon)

1 stick (4 ounces) butter, unsalted

Pinch of salt
½ cup cold water

1. Allow butter to soften to room temperature in a mixing bowl.
2. Whip softened butter with electric mixer until fluffy.
3. Add a little salt and continue to whip at high speed, gradually adding water as you whip.
4. Refrigerate in covered container and use as butter.

LOW-CALORIE MAPLE-FLAVORED SYRUP

(1 cup, 20 calories a tablespoon)

3 ounces pure maple syrup (do not use pancake syrup)
2 teaspoons fructose

1 cup cold water
2 teaspoons arrowroot
¼ teaspoon vanilla

1. Combine all ingredients in saucepan and stir until blended.
2. Heat to simmer and continue simmering until syrup thickens, about 20 minutes.

MAPLE-HONEY SYRUP
*(24 tablespoons,
12 calories a tablespoon)*

2 ounces dark honey
2 teaspoons fructose
1 ounce pure maple syrup (not
   pancake syrup)

2 teaspoons arrowroot
1 cup cold water

1. Combine all ingredients in saucepan.
2. Stir until blended.
3. Heat to simmer and continue to simmer until syrup thickens, about 20 minutes.

MOCK SOUR CREAM
*(40 tablespoon servings,
10 calories each)*

1 pint low-fat cottage cheese
½ cup buttermilk or skim milk
Pinch of salt

1. Combine all ingredients.
2. Blend at high speed until smooth and creamy. Add a scant bit of buttermilk if mixture becomes too dry to blend smoothly.
NOTE: Use as base for various low-calorie dips. Add dried onion or vegetable soup, chives, or other seasoning for flavor.

Desserts

LOW-CAL COTTAGE CHEESE MOUSSE
*(4 servings,
50 calories each)*

1 envelope (4 servings) any
   flavor low-calorie gelatin

½ cup low-fat cottage cheese
1⅓ tablespoons flaked coconut

1. Prepare gelatin according to package instructions.
2. Chill until syrupy.
3. Beat until fluffy.
4. Whip cottage cheese in blender for 20–30 seconds until smooth; add to fluffy gelatin.
5. Beat until well blended.
6. Put in parfait or champagne glasses and top with coconut.

LOW-CALORIE VANILLA ICE CREAM

(8 servings, 90 calories each)

2 egg whites
½ envelope unflavored gelatin
3 tablespoons cold water
13-ounce can evaporated skim milk

½ cup granulated fructose
1½ teaspoons vanilla extract
Pinch of salt

1. Beat egg whites until stiff.
2. Combine gelatin and cold water in saucepan.
3. Wait 1 minute, then heat over low flame until gelatin melts.
4. Remove gelatin from heat; stir in evaporated milk, fructose, vanilla, and salt.
5. Carefully fold gelatin mixture into egg whites and freeze in mixing bowl.
6. Beat twice during freezing.
NOTE: If you have an ice cream maker, use that and follow instructions.

LOW-CALORIE HOT FUDGE SAUCE

(16 tablespoon servings, 20 calories each

2 tablespoons unsweetened cocoa powder
5 tablespoons granulated fructose

1 tablespoon cornstarch
1 cup skim milk
1 teaspoon vanilla extract
Pinch of salt

1. Combine all ingredients in nonstick saucepan.
2. Stir until dissolved.
3. Heat over low flame to simmer, then remove from heat and allow to cool and thicken.

SOFT ICE CREAM

(8 servings, 100 calories each)

2 eggs
2 envelopes unflavored gelatin
¾ cup boiling water

¾ cup granulated fructose
4 teaspoons vanilla extract
1 cup instant nonfat dry milk

1. Break eggs into blender.
2. Sprinkle gelatin on eggs and wait 1 minute.
3. Add boiling water and blend until gelatin dissolves.
4. Add all other ingredients and blend until smooth.
5. Smooth into eight dessert dishes and place in freezer for 15 minutes before serving.

20
The Veggie-thin Omega Diet and Recipes

The Veggie-thin Omega Weight-Loss Diet, like the other Omega diets, can be used "no-choice" by following the menus given. You can also create your own "free-choice" menus by substituting calorie-equivalent vegetarian dishes for the shellfish, fish, fowl, meat, and dairy dishes of the standard Easy-thin Diet or the Gourmet-thin Diet.

In the absence of meat and/or dairy products, high protein is difficult to attain, so some appetite suppression is sacrificed. Commercial high-protein drinks can be used to provide protein; however, limit these to no more than one meal per day.

For the free-choice diet

The recipes for tofu, Roman rice and beans, polenta, the stir-fried dishes, and vegetable dishes that represent nutritionally complete traditional single-dish meals have been provided in chapter 17. Note that the traditional single-dish meals are balanced for protein completeness and are also appropriately high in Omega-3 and Omega-6 EFA as well as other nutrients.

Cauliflower, broccoli, asparagus, vegetable, and watercress soups are appropriate for this diet. Add walnuts, chestnuts, hazelnuts, beechnuts—all high in polyunsaturates and especially Omega-3. The entire repertoire of Chinese vegetable dishes, including chop suey and chow mein, can be used. Serve with small amounts of brown rice. Vegetable stews and ratatouille are other possibilities for menu planning.

Use the northern beans—soy, red, kidney, common, northern, navy—in various warm dishes or with tofu, soups, or vegetable salads. Fruit salads, squash, mushrooms, cucumbers, celery, and carrots make healthful snacks. Eggplant parmesan and various cheese combination dishes are fine for lacto-vegetarians.

Use vegetable bouillon; make French onion soup with or without cheese. Try vegetable and cheese soufflés and casseroles. Cheese fondu can be dipped with raw or *al dente* vegetables. If you are a lacto-ovo-

vegetarian, you will want to add not only skim milk, cheeses, and low-fat cottage cheese but also eggs and various egg dishes such as vegetable quiches to your menus. Many of these are already being used in the Standard Omega Diet. Look in chapter 17 for the recipes.

Dieting rules for the vegetarian dieter

The rules to follow are the same as for people on the Gourmet-thin Diet. Of course, the Omega vegetarian should eat northern whole grains, vegetables, nuts, and seeds. Because of the high fiber content of vegetables, the vegetarian is less in need of a fiber supplement than others.

For a "free-choice" Veggie Diet, follow these guidelines when making up your menus:

- Use stone-ground whole-wheat pastas and flours.
- Balance legumes (peas and beans) and non-legumes (mainly grains— wheat, barley, oats, rice).
- Enjoy low-fat cheeses, milk, and yogurt.
- Have an egg occasionally, as eggs are a good source of complete protein.
- For snacking at any time, use raw celery, radishes, cucumbers, cauliflower, string beans, cherry tomatoes, carrots, turnip slices, lettuce, green peppers, scallions, and zucchini.
- Drink a glass of water during the day any time you feel hunger, but do not drink water near bed time.

I do not recommend an extreme vegetarian diet. You are better assured of fulfilling protein needs with at least some animal protein in your diet— dairy products and eggs at least, if not some meat or fish now and then. Be pragmatic and "listen to your body" to determine *experimentally* what animal protein-to-vegetable ratio makes you feel best.

THE VEGGIE-THIN OMEGA MENU

SUNDAY

		Calories
BREAKFAST	2–4 tablespoons fiber appetizer*	50
	½ cup grapefruit	40
	1 cup hot oatmeal topped with	135
	1 tablespoon toasted sunflower seeds	35
	½ cup skim milk	60
	TOTAL	320
LUNCH	2–4 tablespoons fiber appetizer*	50
	⅓ cup kidney bean salad**	245
	½ cup berries (when in season)	45
	TOTAL	340
MIDAFTERNOON SNACK	1 medium apple or ½ cup skim milk or plain yogurt	60
	TOTAL	60
DINNER	2–4 tablespoons fiber appetizer*	50
	Spinach soufflé**	145
	1 baked tomato	50
	1 small stone-ground whole-wheat muffin with 1 teaspoon butter	120
	½ cup coleslaw with 1 teaspoon Omega mayonnaise	35
	TOTAL	400
EVENING SNACK	½ cup skim milk or cottage cheese	60
	Celery or small carrot sticks	20
	TOTAL	80
	GRAND TOTAL	1200

*Recipe appears on page 29.
**Recipe appears at the end of this chapter.

MONDAY

Calories

BREAKFAST · 2–4 tablespoons fiber appetizer* · 50
½ orange · 40
1 cup Bran Flakes · 140
½ cup skim milk · 60
TOTAL · 290

LUNCH · 2–4 tablespoons fiber appetizer* · 50
2 slices stone-ground whole-grain bread with · 160
3 tablespoons Swiss cheese spread** · 80
Lettuce, tomato, cucumber salad · 20
½ cup skim milk · 60
TOTAL · 370

MIDAFTERNOON · ½ cup skim milk · 60
SNACK · TOTAL · 60

DINNER · 2–4 tablespoons fiber appetizer* · 50
Roman Rice and Beans† · 255
Salad with Omega oil and vinegar dressing · 80
½ slice stone-ground whole-wheat bread · 35
TOTAL · 420

EVENING SNACK · ½ cup skim milk or plain yogurt · 60
Celery and carrot sticks · 20
TOTAL · 80

GRAND TOTAL · 1220

*Recipe appears on page 29.
**Recipe appears at the end of this chapter.
†See recipe section at the end of chapter 17 for recipe.

TUESDAY

			Calories
BREAKFAST	2–4 tablespoons fiber appetizer*		50
	½ grapefruit		40
	Cottage Cheese Grill Maxine††		260
		TOTAL	350
LUNCH	2–4 tablespoons fiber appetizer*		50
	Watercress soup**		90
	½ baked potato, topped with		70
	½ cup low-fat cottage cheese and chives		90
		TOTAL	300
MIDAFTERNOON SNACK	1 medium apple or ½ cup skim milk or plain yogurt		60
		TOTAL	60
DINNER	2–4 tablespoons fiber appetizer*		50
	½ cup fresh fruit or lettuce salad		280
	1 slice stone-ground whole-wheat toast, spread with low-calorie jelly		80
		TOTAL	410
EVENING SNACK	½ cup skim milk or cottage cheese		60
	Celery stalks or carrot sticks		20
		TOTAL	80
		GRAND TOTAL	1200

*Recipe appears on page 29.
**Recipe appears at the end of this chapter.
††See recipe section for Gourmet-thin Diet for recipe.

WEDNESDAY

		Calories
BREAKFAST	2–4 tablespoons fiber appetizer*	50
	½ grapefruit	50
	½ cup Bran Flakes or Shredded Wheat	60
	½ cup skim milk	60
	TOTAL	220
LUNCH	2–4 tablespoons fiber appetizer*	50
	Stuffed pita**	245
	½ cup skim milk	60
	½ cup blueberries or other small fruit	45
	TOTAL	400
MIDAFTERNOON SNACK	½ cup low-fat cottage cheese	30
	½ cup skim milk	60
	TOTAL	90
DINNER	2–4 tablespoons fiber appetizer*	50
	Indian Rice and Beans†	225
	Lettuce and tomato salad with	30
	1 tablespoon red wine dressing	35
	½ cup assorted fruit	70
	TOTAL	410
EVENING SNACK	Small apple	40
	½ ounce low-calorie cheese	50
	TOTAL	90
	GRAND TOTAL	1210

*Recipe appears on page 29.
**Recipe appears at the end of this chapter.
†See recipe section at the end of chapter 17 for recipe.

THURSDAY

		Calories
BREAKFAST	2–4 tablespoons fiber appetizer*	50
	½ grapefruit	50
	French toast**	230
	TOTAL	330
LUNCH	2–4 tablespoons fiber appetizer*	50
	Scrambled eggs with broccoli**	240
	1 slice stone-ground whole-wheat bread	75
	½ cup berries (in season)	35
	TOTAL	400
MIDAFTERNOON SNACK	1 tablespoon sunflower seed kernels	35
	½ cup low-fat yogurt or skim milk	60
	TOTAL	95
DINNER	2–4 tablespoons fiber appetizer*	50
	Ratatouille**	100
	Waldorf salad**	120
	TOTAL	270
EVENING SNACK	1 ounce low-calorie cheese	50
	Small apple	40
	TOTAL	90
	GRAND TOTAL	1185

*Recipe appears on page 29.
**Recipe appears at the end of this chapter.

FRIDAY

		Calories
BREAKFAST	2–4 tablespoons fiber appetizer*	50
	½ orange	40
	1 cup oatmeal	135
	½ cup skim milk	60
	TOTAL	285
LUNCH	2–4 tablespoons fiber appetizer*	50
	1 Middle Eastern Taco**	280
	1 cup bouillon	10
	TOTAL	340
MIDAFTERNOON	½ cup low-fat yogurt	60
SNACK	1 tablespoon chopped walnuts	45
	TOTAL	105
DINNER	2–4 tablespoons fiber appetizer*	50
	Cottage cheese souffle**	210
	Guacamole-stuffed tomato**	110
	TOTAL	370
EVENING SNACK	½ cup skim milk or plain yogurt	60
	4 dried apricot halves	40
	TOTAL	100
	GRAND TOTAL	1200

*Recipe appears on page 29.
**Recipe appears at the end of this chapter.

SATURDAY

			Calories
BREAKFAST	2–4 tablespoons fiber appetizer*		50
	½ grapefruit		50
	Cottage Cheese Grill Maxine††		260
		TOTAL	360
LUNCH	2–4 tablespoons fiber appetizer*		50
	Tabouli**		195
	1 cup French apple yogurt**		65
		TOTAL	310
MIDAFTERNOON SNACK	½ cup skim milk		60
		TOTAL	60
DINNER	2–4 tablespoons fiber appetizer*		50
	Garbanzo and cheese loaf**		330
	Lettuce and tomato salad with		35
	1 tablespoon red wine dressing		25
		TOTAL	440
EVENING SNACK	Cottage cheese mousse†		50
		TOTAL	50
		GRAND TOTAL	1220

*Recipe appears on page 29.
**Recipe appears at the end of this chapter.
†See recipe on page 206.
††See recipe section for Gourmet-thin diet for recipe.

THE VEGGIE-THIN OMEGA DIET RECIPES

Other vegetarian dishes or dishes that can be adapted for vegetarian eating appear in the preceding recipe sections. For salad dressings and low-calorie spreads or sauces, see the recipe section for the Gourmet-thin Omega Diet.

COTTAGE CHEESE SOUFFLÉ

(4 servings, 210 calories each)

4 eggs, separated
¼ cup skim milk
¼ cup stone-ground whole-wheat flour
1 small onion, chopped
1 tablespoon minced fresh parsley

1 teaspoon prepared mustard
¼ teaspoon paprika
1½ teaspoon salt
Pinch of white pepper
2 cups low-fat cottage cheese
Pinch of cream of tartar

1. Beat egg yolks until light yellow.
2. Combine milk and flour into smooth paste and add egg yolks and beat well.
3. Add all remaining ingredients except for egg whites and cream of tartar and beat until smooth.
4. Combine cream of tartar and egg whites; beat until stiff.
5. Carefully fold egg whites into the cheese mixture.
6. Spoon into 1½-quart casserole.
7. Bake in preheated 300-degree oven for 1 hour.
8. Serve immediately.

FRENCH TOAST

1 serving, 230 calories)

1 egg
¼ teaspoon fructose
½ teaspoon vanilla
1½ slices stone-ground whole-wheat or rye bread

1 teaspoon soy or walnut oil
2 tablespoons low-calorie maple syrup (see page 205)

1. Combine and beat together egg, fructose, and vanilla.
2. Soak bread slices
3. Wipe nonstick skillet with oil.
4. Brown egg-soaked bread on both sides over medium heat.
5. Serve with 2 tablespoons low-calorie maple syrup.

GARBANZO AND CHEESE LOAF
(8 servings, 325 calories each)

1 cup chopped onion
3 tablespoons Omega oil
1 cup whole-grain bread
    crumbs
1 cup unsweetened pineapple
    juice
½ cup dry garbanzo beans,
    cooked tender, drained and
    cooled

1 tablespoon miso
¼ cup chopped parsley
½ cup chopped celery
1 egg, beaten
1 cup grated Swiss cheese
1 teaspoon salt
Dash hot sauce
2 pinches of cayenne pepper
Dash of black pepper

1. Sauté onions in 1 tablespoon oil, but do not let brown.
2. Combine bread crumbs and pineapple juice and allow to soak.
3. Coarsely chop or grind the cooked garbanzo beans.
4. Dissolve miso in small amount of hot water.
5. Combine beans and crumb mixture, miso, and remaining ingredients (including remaining oil).
6. Turn the mixture into an oiled loaf pan or small casserole.
7. Bake at 350 degrees for 40 minutes until the edges are browned.
8. Serve hot.

MIDDLE EASTERN TACOS
(10 servings, 280 calories each)

3 cups cooked garbanzo beans
2 cloves garlic, minced
¾ teaspoon ground coriander
½ teaspoon ground cumin
½ cup sesame seeds, toasted
    and ground, or ¼ cup
    sesame butter

2 tablespoons lemon juice
½ teaspoon salt
¼ teaspoon cayenne pepper
10 sesame stone-ground whole-
    wheat pita pockets or 10 stone-
    ground whole-wheat tortillas

1. Combine all ingredients except pita pockets/tortillas and puree. To increase density of spice flavors, let stand at least ½ hour at room temperature after mixing.
2. Fill pockets with bean mixture.
NOTE: For toasty texture, heat filled bread in oven before garnishing, or serve with tortillas—not crisp, but fried until soft. Supply garnishes of yogurt, chopped tomatoes, cucumbers, onion, low-calorie cheese, or shredded lettuce. Let diners assemble their own tacos.

RATATOUILLE

*(8 servings,
100 calories each)*

1 large (1 pound) eggplant
2 medium zucchini
1 large yellow onion
1 green pepper
¼ cup soy oil
3 tomatoes, chopped, or 5
   tablespoons tomato paste
   and 3 tablespoons water

1 teaspoon salt
⅛ teaspoon pepper
½ teaspoon oregano
½ teaspoon basil
½ clove garlic, minced

1. Dice eggplant into 1″ cubes, slice zucchini in ½″ rounds, chop onion coarsely, and cut green peppers into 1″ squares.
2. In heavy-bottomed saucepan, sauté onions, garlic, and green pepper in oil until soft.
3. Stir in eggplant and zucchini and sauté a few more minutes.
4. Add tomato and seasonings.
5. Cover and simmer gently for about 30 minutes, until all vegetables are well cooked.
6. Uncover and turn up heat to evaporate some of the liquid.
7. Serve hot.

SCRAMBLED EGGS WITH BROCCOLI

*(2 servings,
250 calories each)*

4 eggs
¼ cup skim milk
¼ teaspoon salt
Dash of paprika
Dash of Tabasco sauce

½ cup chopped and drained
   cooked broccoli
½ cup low-fat cottage cheese
½ teaspoon soy or walnut oil

1. Lightly beat eggs in medium bowl.
2. Add milk, salt, paprika, and Tabasco.
3. Stir in broccoli and cottage cheese.
4. Wipe medium nonstick skillet with ½ teaspoon oil.
5. Pour egg mixture into skillet.
6. Cook over low heat, stirring occasionally, until eggs are set but still moist.
7. Serve immediately.

SPINACH SOUFFLÉ

*(8 servings,
80 calories each)*

20 ounces fresh chopped or 2
   10-ounce packages frozen
   chopped spinach, defrosted
4 eggs
1 cup evaporated milk

½ teaspoon onion salt
¼ teaspoon grated nutmeg
2 tablespoons grated Romano
   cheese

1. Combine spinach, eggs, milk, onion salt, and nutmeg in a blender.
2. Blend at medium speed.
3. Pour into a 1-quart baking dish.
4. Sprinkle top with grated cheese.
5. Bake in preheated 350-degree oven 1 hour or more, until center is set.
6. Serve immediately.

TABOULI

*(8 servings,
200 calories each)*

1½ cups whole northern wheat,
   uncooked
3 cups vegetable stock or water
1 teaspoon salt
Pepper to taste
½ cup cooked white northern
   beans
2 tomatoes, chopped
2 tablespoons soy or walnut oil

1 clove garlic, minced
2 tablespoons chopped chives or
   scallions
2 tablespoons fresh chopped mint
   leaves
1¼ cups chopped parsley
Lettuce
Juice of three lemons

1. Crack wheat seeds by running them in the blender for 5 seconds.
2. Bring stock or water to boil, adding salt and pepper.
3. Add cracked wheat slowly to boiling water.
4. Boil for 5 minutes longer.
5. Remove from heat, cover tightly, and set aside for 2 hours. (NOTE: If you use bulgur wheat, just bring to a boil, cover and set aside for 1 hour.)
6. Remove excess water from grain by shaking cooked wheat in a strainer, or squeeze wheat with hands.
7. Chill the grain.
8. Toss cool grain thoroughly with the remaining ingredients, except lettuce.
9. Season further to taste and serve on a bed of lettuce.

STUFFED PITA

(1 serving, 240 calories)

½ cup chopped asparagus, green beans, or broccoli
½ cup chopped tomato
1 tablespoon alfalfa sprouts
1 teaspoon chopped shallots

Cayenne pepper to taste
½ teaspoon basil
½ 7" pita bread,
¼ cup coarsely grated sharp cheddar cheese

1. Steam green vegetables until crisp-tender.
2. Mix steamed vegetables with tomato, sprouts, shallots, and seasoning in medium bowl.
3. Spoon vegetables into pita pocket.
4. Spread cheese over vegetable surface and heat in 350-degree oven until cheese melts.
5. Serve immediately.

VEGETABLE SALAD

(main dish, 1 serving, 130 calories)

1 cup shredded lettuce
½ cup alfalfa sprouts
½ cup chopped celery
¼ cup chopped scallions

½ cup chopped broccoli flowerets and stalks
¼ cup cooked soybeans

1. Toss all ingredients together.
2. Add low-calorie salad dressing.

GUACAMOLE-STUFFED TOMATO

(4 servings, 115 calories each)

4 tomatoes, peeled and hollowed (invert for 20 minutes to drain)
1 tablespoon finely chopped onion
Pulp from 1 tomato

1 teaspoon minced pickled jalapeno pepper
1 ripe avocado, pared and mashed with fork
2 tablespoons lemon juice
½ teaspoon salt

1. While the tomatoes drain, mix other ingredients together.
2. Spoon about ¼ cup guacamole mixture into each hollowed tomato.
3. Adjust seasoning, and serve on a bed of lettuce.

KIDNEY BEAN SALAD

*(8 servings,
245 calories each)*

1 cup dry kidney beans, cooked
  and drained
1 green pepper, chopped
½ cup chopped onions or
  scallions
1 teaspoon crushed garlic
½ cup soy or walnut oil
¼ cup wine vinegar
1 cup chopped cucumber
⅛ teaspoon paprika

1 teaspoon honey
1 tablespoon tomato catsup
1 cup chopped celery
¼ teaspoon salt
1 teaspoon Worcestershire sauce
2 tablespoons minced fresh
  parsley
Dash of hot sauce
1 cup plain yogurt
¼ cup nonfat dry powdered milk

1. Combine cooked beans, green pepper, onions or scallions, and garlic.
2. Make a salad dressing by combining oil, wine vinegar, and the remaining ingredients, except for the yogurt and milk powder.
3. Pour the dressing over the bean mixture and toss gently.
4. Refrigerate this marinade at least 1 hour.
5. Combine the yogurt and powdered milk.
6. Just before serving, stir in the yogurt-milk powder mixture. Serve on a bed of lettuce.

WALDORF SALAD

*(6 servings,
130 calories each)*

1 cup diced celery
1 cup white seedless grapes
¾ cup low-calorie Omega
  mayonnaise (see page 200)

1 cup diced apples
½ cup chopped walnuts
12 lettuce leaves

1. Combine all ingredients except lettuce.
2. Serve, arranging salad on 2 lettuce leaves for each serving.

WATERCRESS SOUP

*(2 servings,
100 calories each)*

1 bunch watercress, washed and
  trimmed
1 envelope instant onion broth
  or bouillon mix

1 cup low-fat yogurt
Salt and pepper to taste
1 cup water
2 thin slices lemon

1. Puree all ingredients except water and lemon.
2. Pour into saucepan; add water. Bring just to boiling point, stirring frequently.

3. Spoon into soup bowls and float a slice of lemon on each serving.
4. Serve hot and garnish with a spray of watercress.
NOTE: This soup can also be made with broccoli, cabbage, spinach, Swiss chard, or cauliflower instead of watercress.

BLACK BEAN SOUP

(9 1-cup servings, 225 calories each)

1½ cups black turtle beans
1½ quarts vegetable stock or water
2 tablespoons soy or walnut oil
2 stalks celery, chopped
1 carrot, chopped
1 potato, chopped
1 bay leaf
¼ teaspoon savory

1 clove garlic, minced
1 teaspoon oregano
2½ tablespoons dry red wine
2 teaspoons salt
⅛ teaspoon pepper
Juice of one lemon
1 onion, chopped
2 eggs, hard-boiled
½ lemon, thinly sliced

1. Wash beans and soak them overnight in 4 cups of water.
2. Drain beans, put in a pressure cooker with 1½ quarts of water or stock and 1 tablespoon oil (to prevent foaming).
3. Pressure cook at 15 pounds pressure for 15 minutes.
4. Reduce pressure gradually.
5. Sauté celery, carrots, and potatoes in 1 tablespoon oil.
6. Add vegetables, garlic, and herbs to beans.
7. Bring soup to a boil then lower heat to simmer until done.
8. Cool slightly and remove bay leaf.
9. Pour 1½ cups soup into blender and process until smooth.
10. Transfer processed soup to 2-quart bowl and repeat until all soup is processed.
11. Pour soup back into saucepan.
12. Add wine, salt, and pepper and bring to a broil.
13. Reduce heat to simmer for 5 minutes.
14. Stir in lemon juice.
15. Pour soup into bowls; garnish with chopped egg, chopped onion, and lemon slices. Serve hot with a little sherry.
NOTE: The gas-producing component of beans is eliminated with the overnight soaking and cooking the beans until very tender.

FRENCH APPLE YOGURT

3 cups diced or sliced apples
2 cups plain yogurt
1 teaspoon vanilla

½ teaspoon cinnamon
1 teaspoon fructose, if apples are
tart

1. Cook apples in ½ cup water 5–10 minutes, until soft.
2. Reserve 1 cup of apples and put rest in blender.
3. Add 1 cup yogurt, vanilla, cinnamon, and fructose.
4. Blend briefly. Add reserved apples and remaining yogurt. Mix all ingredients together.
5. Serve chilled.

SWISS CHEESE SPREAD

½ cup grated Swiss cheese
¼ cup chopped green pepper
1 tablespoon low-calorie Omega
mayonnaise (see page 200)

½ cup low-fat cottage cheese
½ teaspoon dill weed
Salt and pepper to taste

1. Mix all ingredients together.
2. Refrigerate until ready to serve.
3. Add hard-boiled egg, chives, parsley, ½ teaspoon paprika, or ¼ teaspoon mustard powder as a garnish, or mix into spread to change flavor or texture.

21
The Omega
Antiallergy Diet

Many of the people who participated in my study of the Omega-3 EFA suffered immune problems, including food allergies. The food allergies revealed themselves as diarrhea, breathing difficulties, hives, nausea, flushing, quickened heartbeat, and headaches within a few hours after eating the offending food(s). However, when the symptoms were not violent, many of the victims did not realize they'd suffered allergic reactions provoked by foods that were eaten so regularly that their correlation with illness was difficult to trace. Keeping a "food diary" and noting daily symptoms can sometimes uncover the troublemakers. Another common approach is to undertake lengthy and expensive tests for food allergens.

But there is another way: Follow the Omega Standard Diet, with or without the Omega Supplement Program, to see if this eliminates the problem over a period of a few months. If not, the immune system may be so overwhelmed by the food allergens that you cannot respond to any therapy until the allergens have been identified and removed from your diet for a period of several months. To achieve this identification and removal of the allergens, try either the Omega chemical sensitivity diet or the Omega food elimination diets, which are explained in this section.

Common food allergies and how to test for them

Food allergies are everywhere. The most common food allergens include:

Beans	Fish	Peas
Chocolate	Garlic	Shellfish
Citrus fruits	Milk	Tomato
Corn	Nuts	Wheat
Eggs	Onions	Yeast

225

All products containing one or more of these ingredients, even in small quantities, can cause allergic reactions from wheezing to rashes. Arthritics tend to be sensitive to the nightshades—the small-seed plants such as tomatoes, eggplant, peppers, and potatoes, all of which contain solanine, a steroidal compound. Among the inorganic food additives many people are sensitive to:

- Monosodium glutamate—often used in Chinese cooking and prepared foods
- Nitrates and nitrites—found in luncheon meats, hot dogs, ham, and bacon
- Sulfites—used to keep greens "fresh" and sometimes added to the vegetables in salads bars

To identify the offending food or substance, the common allergens listed above and any other suspected foods must be eliminated from the diet for starters. No foods or fluids may be consumed other than those specified in the elimination diet (see below) for a period of two weeks. This also rules out eating in restaurants, since you must know or be able to determine the exact composition of all dishes in all meals. Read labels to be certain of the purity of the products used. For example, ordinary rye bread contains some wheat flour.

If no improvement occurs after two weeks on the first elimination diet, then try a different group of foods in the second elimination diet for another two-week period.

When symptoms are relieved, you add new foods to the diet and eat them regularly in large amounts for at least three days to see which provokes an adverse reaction.

Wheat (gluten) and milk—common allergens

The procedure just described will detect milk and gluten (the characteristic protein found in all cereals) sensitivities, both of which are very common. Both can produce skin rashes and gastrointestinal discomfort (celiac disease). I think another form of this allergy—"a cerebral allergic reaction"—may be a major contributor to mental illnesses.

If a gluten or gluten-milk sensitivity is discovered through the test diets, a gluten-free or gluten-and-milk-free diet is recommended. Food allergy management can be quite complex. If you have an allergy, it is best to adjust your diet to eliminate the food allergens. However, after several months on the Omega program many people find that their sensitivity to a particular food disappears as their immune systems return to normal. But remember: *Do not try any diet without first discussing it with your physician.*

Omega chemical-sensitivity diet for severe cases

The most effective dietary method for detecting a food allergy is use of the chemical diet, a nutritive formula in which all food components are broken down to their elemental nonallergenic nutritive forms. This is the diet that is used to prepare people for gastrointestinal surgery. This nutritionally complete liquid diet is related to the liquid weight-loss diets and, although it is available through druggists, should be used only under the guidance of a physician. One commercially available liquid nonallergenic diet is Vivonex. Many people have lived for a number of years sustained by such diets alone.

The liquid foods available through most local druggists can be "Omegafied" by adding Omega oils—about one to three tablespoons of soybean or other oil for every 2,000 calories of liquid drink. The fiber "appetizer" (see page 29 for the standard recipe) should be taken along with the drink for its best effect, but you should first test for possible allergenic factors in the soy oil and fibers themselves. This is done in the following way:

1. Start the Vivonex or equivalent with no added oil or fiber for a week.
2. Introduce an Omega oil, switching between soy, walnut, and sunflower every five days.
3. Start with no fiber at all.
4. After five days, introduce either pectin, psyllium seed, or miller's bran.
5. After five more days, switch to another fiber.
6. Note any adverse reactions.
7. Note any positive benefits.

How to test for food allergies

It may take a minimum of two weeks to see improvement. If improvement is noted, start a "provocation routine" by supplanting about half the chemical liquid diet with a specific group, three times a day for three days.

Begin with Diet #1 in the table below—a vegetable, lamb, and rice diet. If your trouble does not disappear in one week, then go on to Diet #2 for the following two weeks, and so forth. If you experience a reaction to a particular food or food group, go directly to one of the numbered diets that does not contain the suspect foods. Your symptoms should abate. You can then guess which food causes your food sensitivity. Try to provoke symptoms by reincluding the food as a double check.

Food Allergy Elimination Diets

Foodstuff	Diet #1 (No beef, pork, fowl, rye, corn, wheat, or milk)	Diet #2 (No beef, lamb, rice, wheat, or milk)	Diet #3 (No lamb, fowl, rye, rice, corn, wheat, or milk)	Diet #4 (Nothing but milk)
Cereal	rice products	corn products	none	none
Vegetables	lettuce, beets, spinach, artichokes, carrots	corn, tomatoes, peas, squash, asparagus, string beans	lima beans, string beans, tomatoes, potatoes (white and sweet)	none
Meat	lamb	chicken, ham	beef, bacon	none
Flour	rice	corn, 100% rye (ordinary rye contains wheat)	lima beans, soybeans, potato	none
Fruit	lemons, pears, grapefruit	peaches, prunes, apricots, pineapple	grapefruit, peaches, lemons, apricots	none
Fat	walnut oil	linseed oil	soy	none
Beverage	tea, lemonade, black coffee	spring water	juice from approved fruits, black coffee, tea	none
Miscellaneous	tapioca, cane sugar, gelatin, olives, salt	corn syrup, gelatin, salt	tapioca, honey, gelatin, olives, salt	none
Milk	none	none	none	only (no other dairy products)

22
The Omega Mother-Infant Diet

Both mothers and fathers need good nutrition to ensure healthy babies. If the prospective mother and father were nutritionally fit before conception, no other dietary controls would be necessary. Instead, most live on the Great American Experimental Diet. Ideally, to normalize the germ plasm that forms the prospective embryo, both the mother- and father-to-be should go on the Standard Omega Diet at least six months before conception. The prospective mother, at least, should then continue to follow the Omega nutrition and exercise regimen, augmenting meal size through additional protein intake during pregnancy and the nursing period. If she is of average build, she should gain about three pounds each month for a total of about twenty-five pounds. (She should not follow a weight-reduction diet during pregnancy.)

Increasing food intake

During pregnancy, an expectant mother's calorie and essential nutrient intake should be increased about 10 to 15 percent above normal. For example, if you usually need about 2,500 calories a day, increase your daily intake by 250 to 300 calories.

During nursing, an additional 10 to 15 percent over and above the pregnancy level is best. Nursing mothers need anywhere from 500 to 1,000 calories more than their prepregnancy quota.

Both expectant and nursing mothers should get their additional calories mainly from fish and chicken protein. Protein should be eaten to supply the additional nutritional needs of the growing fetus in utero, and of the infant during breast-feeding. Barring special problems, most physicians also recommend taking a one-a-day multivitamin/multimineral supplement during pregnancy. There are several commercial formulas designed for the expectant mother. Some of these provide megadoses of vitamin B_6, which are not necessary if the mother's diet includes sufficient Omega oils.

Special diets may cause some problems

From the time of conception on, a prospective mother suffering a disease should be treated with dietary supplements. How many and what kind is a complex problem; the supplemental program that is best for the mother's health may not be best for the fetus. For example, a pregnant woman on megavitamins or mega-oils may find that her regimen controls her arthritis during pregnancy but should realize it might cause problems for the developing embryo. While her general health should be as good as possible, the fetus does not have arthritis and may be subject to adverse effects caused by supplement levels kept high enough to help the mother. Similar problems are encountered by diabetic women during pregnancy.

Probably the best compromise in cases like this is to decrease the mother's therapeutic nutritional supplements to the lowest possible level that still gives a minimum of control over the mother's illness. Problems this complex must, of course, be worked out in consultation with your professional health advisers.

Breast-feeding

If possible, the new mother should breast-feed her baby and follow the Standard Omega Diet, augmented for calories and with the supplements mentioned. Breast-feeding should continue for at least six months, and preferably for up to the first two years of a baby's life. The demand for breast-feeding will decrease after six months, as the infant's diet comes to include solid food. Breast-feeding is extremely beneficial to infants because, assuming that the mother is eating properly, there is an ideal Omega balance in the mother's milk. Antibodies carried in human milk also increase disease resistance in the newborn. Additionally, the psychological benefits for mother and baby gained from nursing should not be underestimated.

Omega infant formula

If breast-feeding is impossible, the best alternative is to use a wet nurse who is on the Standard Omega Diet. Failing this, resort to an infant formula using soybean oil, cod liver oil, or similar high Omega-3/Omega-6 EFA, although this alternative is not comparable to breast-feeding. One brand of acceptable infant formula is Soylac. It uses nonhydrogenated soy oil as the source of Omega EFA.

THE OMEGA BABY AND TODDLER DIET

When your baby starts on solid food, its diet should be "Omegafied" by using only baby foods that are low in sugar, hydrogenated oils, and southern oils. Nonhydrogenated Omega oils—cod liver, soy, wheat germ, walnut, or linseed oil—are the preferred sources of EFA in the diet. You can make your own baby food, buy high-Omega baby foods, or add Omega oils to commercially available foods. Starting your baby on the right foods and encouraging your baby to develop a taste for high-Omega and high-fiber foods will give him or her a good start for a lifetime.

Starting your baby on solid foods

Solid foods should be started no earlier than six months of age, to avoid crowding out milk or provoking sensitivities to foods that a baby's immature digestive system is not yet ready to handle. Between six and ten months, you may gradually introduce solids. To be on the safe side, especially if there are allergies in the family, offer the baby only one bite or one-half teaspoon of a new food the first day, slowly increasing the amount during the next few days. Don't introduce more than one new food over a five-day period. In that way you can make sure that each new item is well tolerated.

At one year, the baby will be getting about a quart of breast or bottled milk daily, plus at least three meals and several snacks. Good "starter" foods are oatmeal, applesauce and other cooked fruits, and mashed, steamed vegetables such as carrots, beets, yams, and squash. When your baby is nine to ten months of age, you can add cooked egg yolk, then gradually introduce cooked egg white as well. Cottage cheese usually is accepted well, and at this time you can add small pieces of fish, fowl, or lamb. (Lamb liver is an especially good source of iron.)

Most of these foods come from the family fare. Ideally, they should be prepared for the baby without sugar and salt. The infant's natural taste for sweets is well satisfied by lactose (milk sugar) in milk and by natural sweet fruits and vegetables. Mothers can save their children from a losing battle with sugar cravings later on by understanding this and sticking firmly to the principle of no sweets and no added sweetening in baby's food. Added salt is not required either, since milk and other foods provide plenty of natural salt for the baby's sodium needs.

Growing strong and healthy

The one-year-old can eat a variety of food from the family's Standard Omega-3 Diet as long as the food is mashed or cut into small pieces. Of course, only butter and unhydrogenated oil such as walnut, soy, and linseed should be used in preparing the food. Cod liver or fish oil—five to ten drops by dropper or teaspoon—should be given. Fresh orange juice and pureed fruits are usually a welcome addition to baby's diet. You can dissolve vitamin C powder without a noticeable flavor change whenever you want to give your baby extra vitamin C.

By the time the baby has four molars at twelve to eighteen months of age and can chew reasonably well, steamed vegetables should be served *al dente*—firm instead of mushy—and raw fruits can be added to the diet. **Warning:** Peanuts and other nuts are too easy to choke on at this age, but Omega nut butters are a valuable food for the baby.

By the time the child is three and has all twenty baby teeth, raw vegetables and fresh unsalted nuts and seeds—e.g., walnuts, almonds, chestnuts, hazel nuts, sunflower seeds, and pumpkin seeds—will be a much enjoyed part of the day's meals and snacks. At this age, your child most likely will be eating most of the foods in the family's Standard Omega-3 Diet.

Fiber as part of your baby's diet

In general, ample fiber intake is important not only for the baby's overall health but for bowel training, because sufficient dietary fiber prevents constipation. As the baby gradually adds the natural fiber from vegetables, whole-grain cereals, beans, and fruit to its daily intake, constipation in the form of dry, hard stools that are difficult to pass should not be a problem. If it is, small amounts of unprocessed bran given with pureed fruit or yogurt or added to cereals should allow formation of well-shaped bowel movements that are passed effortlessly.

Omega Baby Foods

When commercially prepared infant and toddler foods are used, ideally they should be:

- Low in added sugar or other sweeteners
- Low in added salt
- Low in hydrogenated oils
- Adequate in unhydrogenated Omega-3 and Omega-6 oils
- High in fiber

23

Longevity and the Omega Antiaging Diet

Most microscopic one-celled life forms—bacteria, yeast, algae, and protozoa—never die of old age. They live forever unless stopped by predators, starvation, or accidents. But we higher life forms are so successful at survival that nature must kill us off internally, by a genetic aging program, so that there will be room for new variations. We die because we are part of a program of biologically planned obsolescence.

Accidents to genetic material are inherent in the nature of chemistry, whether caused by radiation, free radical oxidative attack, chemicals, or other cell-destroying activities. But the one-celled organism that can live forever and the multi-celled organisms that cannot both have a common gene that produces an enzyme to repair accumulating genetic abnormalities. Just as the regular immune system destroys abnormal cells in the body, so the "immortality gene" serves as a kind of immune system for the genetic material, destroying abnormal genes.

Suppression of this genetic repair immune system gradually leads to abnormal genes that produce distorted enzymes or "aging proteins," which cause body functions to deteriorate. Cells and tissues weaken, speeding the final breakdown—death.

The immortal cell types and our own mortal system differ primarily in the effectiveness of the gene-repairing system—the immortality gene. Some evidence suggests that it may be blocked by a protein—an aging protein. If so, and if we could make an antibody to that protein—an antiaging antibody—we would have a vaccine against aging.

Cancer cells—immortals that do not need EFA/prostaglandins

When our own normal cells are transformed into aberrant cells, such as cancer cells, they become immortal and lose their normal prostaglandin responses and dependence on the essential fatty acids that serve as cell "civilizing" regulators. Cancer cells are not cooperative members of the whole organism, responsive to the tissue-level regulatory EFA. They behave like one-celled life forms and do not die naturally, simply replicating over and over again. They must be cut away surgically or killed through radiation or other therapy if they are not to overwhelm the system.

Premature aging can be triggered by a deficiency in EFA

Two rare genetic disorders produce the full range of aging problems in early childhood. In the diseases progeria and xeroderma pigmentosa, the afflicted children—who often die before they reach their teens—look wizened and old, suffer baldness, arthritis, aging spots, heart disease, strokes, and EFA-centered malnutrition: all signs of aging.

In normal aging, the gradual diminution of the enzymes that run the EFA/prostaglandin regulatory system brings on an array of disorders. Our modern malnutrition speeds and exaggerates the normal course of aging, causing an *aging disease*. If we can keep our EFA prostaglandin machinery and its cofactors from slowing, we can also slow or reverse abnormal aging. EFA can be a step toward the fountain of youth, and methods already used to extend our life-span may be enhanced by stimulating our EFA/prostaglandin mechanisms.

Aging and the need for EFA

It has been hard to identify the specific gene system, deteriorating enzymes, or aging patterns that eventually kill us. The same problem is true in the field of nutrition where a variety of theories cast blame on many different factors for our nutritional ill health:

Antinutritional factors	Favorable nutritional factors
Sugar	Polyunsaturated EFA
Cholesterol	Selenium
Saturated fats	Fiber
Stress	Antioxidants
	Vitamins

Aging can be accelerated by disrupting the EFA/prostaglandin system and blocking antioxidants. Many of the ailments associated with aging are hard to distinguish from EFA malnutrition. They are:

Dry skin	Tinnitus
Cardiovascular ailments	Glaucoma
Arthritis	Weakened immune system

Omega Rats Live Longer

A breed of notoriously short-lived immune-deficient mice showed significantly longer survival when given supplements of fish oil Omega-3 EFA. In other experiments, rats given all required nutrients but kept underfed have survived about 50 percent longer than average when Omega-3 EFA was provided.

Underfeeding stimulates important enzymes that desaturate the essential fatty acids, while aging decreases this activity. It has been discovered that rats live longer when given supplements of the antioxidants selenium and vitamin E, which protect the EFA.

The prospect of staying half-starved in order to live longer has little appeal for most of us. A better way to spur our EFA/prostaglandin apparatus is to follow the Omega regimen, making use of important antioxidants and EFA as well as aerobic exercise and stress reduction.

Aging and two kinds of malnutrition

Two kinds of malnutrition exist:

1. Dietary—resulting when nutrients are lacking
2. Metabolic—resulting when nutrients are available but the body's ability to use them is impaired, as in aging

Aging tends to shut down metabolic efficiency so that older people who are additionally suffering dietary malnutrition will be in double jeopardy. A dietary lack of nutrients accelerates the rate of aging and that in turn worsens metabolic malnutrition as digestion, absorption, and utilization of nutrients decline, thus begetting a vicious circle.

In dietary deficiency, the blood levels of nutrients are usually low, while in metabolic malnutrition, blood levels may be normal or even high. But the nutrients don't reach the cells, so the tissues are starved. In either situation, nutrient supplements should be used—in dietary and aging deficiency to fill the empty reservoirs, and in metabolic deficiency to provide a flood of nutrients to help overcome metabolic blocks to their utilization.

With aging there is a declining requirement for calories; when calorie needs fall below 1,500 calories per day, the distribution of nutrients in foods makes it very difficult to obtain even a minimum daily requirement (the RDA). For this reason, because of their metabolic deficiency, and due to the damaging effect of the typical American diet, older people should augment their nutrition with supplements to make sure they get needed nutrients. The RDA for older people is not necessarily that recommended by the Nutrition Council for healthy adults.

Fatty acids and enzymes

Since the enzymes that process essential fatty acids diminish with age, adding oils to the diet may be especially helpful. Fish oils contain EPA and DHA Omega-3 fatty acids, which elderly people, who have fewer needed enzymes, have trouble making from linseed oil. So increase your fish consumption as you get older. By experimenting with varying ratios of linseed and fish oil you can discover what combination is best for you.

Life extension—it is possible

Here are four ways to help fight aging:

1. Follow the Standard Omega Diet.
2. Take a complete one-a-day multivitamin-multimineral supplement that includes the antioxidants—vitamin pro-A (beta-carotene), vitamin C, and vitamin E, selenium, and cysteine-methionine.
3. Take a premeal fiber "appetizer" three times a day. (Add flaxseed as a combined source of fiber and EFA.)
4. Participate in a program of aerobic exercise suitable to your strength and health.

Within these guidelines, try different ratios in the amounts of protein to carbohydrate to oils over a three-week period and note your reactions. Keep a diary, it will help you find your optimum diet. Here is how to set up a chart:

Chart Your Reaction

Time	Protein	Carbohydrates	Oils	Reaction
Day 1				
Day 2				
Day 3				

High-protein meals are often used as supplemental diets before surgery or to give debilitated people a boost. Avoid high-protein diets, however, if you have liver and kidney disease, because the metabolizing of proteins places an additional burden on these organs. With illness or aging, a trial of the Omega Standard or Gourmet-thin diet with calories adjusted upward may prove to be helpful.

Interestingly, there are plant forms and possibly some fish that can switch between the immortal and mortal (aging) state, depending on environmental triggers and induced mutations. Man himself may be only a few mutations away from immortality. He may even discover an antiaging vaccine. In the meantime, we can fight our metabolic and dietary malnutrition with the nutritionally complete and highly synergistic Omega Diet and Omega Supplement Program.

24

Beware
The Great American
Experimental Diet

The average American diet is deficient in a multitude of interacting nutrients and loaded with antinutrients. Just as it took more than a century for scientists and physicians to learn to diagnose and treat the B-vitamin deficiency diseases beriberi and pellagra, so the more nutritionally complex diseases we face today have until now also eluded identification.

Through the study of human nutritional needs, a new picture of health and disease emerges. Although a vast quantity of food is available, there is a shocking increase in many illnesses, an epidemic of the modernization diseases. While these diseases are treated today as distinct and unrelated they seem actually to be alternative symptomatic forms of a synergistic malnutrition.

Modern malnutrition is the enemy

The Standard Omega Diet presented in this book is the first complete nutritional program. It is a universal diet. Similarly, the Omega Supplement Program constitutes the first *complete* supplemental regimen providing the full synergistic benefits of all essential nutrients and their powerful interactions.

Consumer beware

There are risks to everything. In any large group there is always a chance that someone will be adversely affected by a particular diet or supplement, but the relative risk-to-benefit ratio of the Omega program is excellent, especially if you start at RDA levels and work up to higher levels gradually every few days. I think the real danger lies in continuing to eat the average American diet, which should be regarded as the *real* experiment—the Great American Experimental Diet—interactively modified, untested, and unproven.

Don't get trapped in expensive supplement programs. The Omega program should cost you no more than a few pennies to fifty cents a day, unless you are taking—and need—very large amounts of expensive fish oils and megavitamins for a short period of time. Work out your own optimum dose for the various meganutrients. Follow the guidelines given in this book and shop for your nutrients at your local nutrition store, the nutrition center in your supermarket, or via mail order catalogs from reliable firms.

More and more physicians are treating themselves with nutritional supplements, even if they won't prescribe this "orthotherapy" for their patients. Although standards of practice are still being established, Appendix A lists some of the more reputable associations of reform nutritionists and reform physicians—"orthotherapists"—who provide the kind of therapy discussed in this book. Some of them are now using linseed oil supplements as the result of the work reported here. There are also guidelines for how to find reputable orthodox "allotherapists" (orthodox medical physicians), and a list of other resources to which you can turn.

Glossary

Acne: A disease of the sebaceous (oil) glands that can lead to inflammation of the skin.

Aerobic exercise: Any physical activity performed in excess of ten minutes that requires an increased supply of oxygen and uses large muscle groups in continuous motion. Aerobic exercises include swimming, jogging, jumping rope, jazz or aerobic dancing, brisk walking.

Aging disease: Premature aging.

Alopecia: Hair loss, baldness.

Alpha linolenic acid: An Omega-3 fatty acid that cannot be made by the human body. It is polyunsaturated and made by marine plants and animals and cold-climate terrestrial plants—nuts, cereals, and seeds. The plant food that has the highest proportion of alpha linolenic acid is linseed oil.

Amenorrhea: Absence of menstrual periods.

Amino acids: The building blocks of protein used to form hair, skin, and other body tissues.

Anemia: A deficiency of hemoglobin in red blood cells, which may as a consequence also be reduced in number and size. The red blood cells carry oxygen in the blood.

Angina: Chest pain that occurs after mild to vigorous exercise or excitement. It is caused by reduced blood supply to the heart, usually as a result of an obstruction of the arteries.

Anosmia: Loss of smell.

Antinutrient: A dietary component that either inhibits the action of essential nutrients or increases the need for them.

Antioxidant: A compound that protects other compounds and tissues from reacting with oxygen.

Aorta: The large artery leaving the left ventricle of the heart.

Arachidonic acid: An Omega-6 essential fatty acid found in milk, meat, and organ meats.

Artery: A blood vessel that supplies blood, oxygen, and nutrients to the tissues of the body.

Arteriosclerosis: Hardening of the arteries.

Atherosclerosis: Deposits of cholesterol and fat-containing plaques in the lining of the arteries.

Autism: An early childhood disorder producing extreme withdrawal and lack of responsiveness; there is often a strong object orientation.

Bacteria: Microscopic one-celled plants without green coloring matter.

Benign: Not malignant, not harmful.

Beriberi: A disease that develops when thiamine is inadequate in the diet.

Beta carotene (pro-vitamin A): A precursor of vitamin A found in plant foods such as carrots and dark green leafy vegetables.

Brown adipose tissue (BAT): A type of fat that maintains body temperature by burning off calories. Brown fat.

Bursitis: An inflammation of the membranes of the bursa, sacs that protect tendons where they meet with friction, such as at the joints. "Tennis elbow" is a common form of bursitis.

Caffeine: A stimulant found in coffee, tea, and many foods, including chocolate.

Calorie: A measurement of heat. A nutritional measurement referring to the quantity of energy contained in food.

Cancer: Cells or groups of cells that behave in a disorderly way, growing wildly.

Capillary: One of the tiny blood vessels connecting arteries and veins through which oxygen and nutrients are released to the tissues and cell waste products are accepted for eventual elimination.

Carbohydrate: The starches and sugars in the diet. Many starches are complex carbohydrates; most sugars are simple carbohydrates.

Carcinogen: Any of a large variety of agents inducing cancer.

Cardiovascular disease: A disease of the heart and blood vessels, usually caused by the accumulation of atherosclerotic plaque.

Carotene: The precursor form of provitamin A found in plants.

Carpal tunnel syndrome: Inflammation of the tendon of the wrist running through the carpal tunnel to the fingers.

Cellulose: A type of dietary fiber.

Chelate: An organic compound with several small groups or "claws" (*chelate* means "claws") that can enfold and bind a metal atom such as calcium, zinc, or iron.

Cholesterol: A type of steroid fat found in many foods that come from animals. It is also produced by the human body. Cholesterol is needed for the production of some hormones, vitamin D, and for healthy nerves and cells. Excessive cholesterol has been linked with several diseases, including cardiovascular diseases and atherosclerosis.

Collagen: The supportive protein substance that keeps cells together; a cellular protein tissue.

Conutrients: Essential nutrients that interact with each other in the body so that the sum of their activities is greater than merely the cumulative individual effects.

Cuticle: The outer covering of the hair and the thin layer of tough skin that covers the base of the nail.

Depression: Extreme and prolonged feelings of melancholy; the "blues."

Dermatitis: Inflammation of the skin.

Dermis: The lower level of the skin.

Deoxyribonucleic acid (DNA): The material in the cell that contains the genetic code.

Diabetes: A disease in which the body is unable to burn its intake of sugars, starches, and other carbohydrates because of either inadequate insulin or a block in the use of insulin.

Diuretic: A substance that increases the flow of urine.

Diverticulitis: An inflammation of the large bowel in which small fingerlike pouches of its lining became irritated and inflamed.

Docosahexaenoic acid (DHA): An essential fatty acid of the Omega-3 family, especially rich in fish and especially cold-water fish.

Double bond: A region of unsaturation.

Dyspareunia: Painful intercourse.

Eczema: The name applied to rough, red skin rashes occurring in patches. It may itch or burn, swell or ooze, often in response to an allergy.

Edema: Swelling of body tissues as a result of being water-logged.

Enzyme: A protein catalyst that accelerates reactions without being changed itself.

Essential fatty acid (EFA): A fatty acid that the body cannot make, with two or more regions of unsaturation.

Esophagus: The passageway from the throat to the stomach.

Estrogen: A female steroid hormone produced and secreted by the ovaries. It is also present in the adrenal cortex, adipose tissue, and other tissues that take over production after menopause.

Fiber: A generic term for the many plant constituents that are not digestible by humans and so pass through the digestive system without being absorbed or broken down.

"Flaky paint" dermatitis: Flaking of the forearms and legs caused by very dry skin.

Formication: The sensation of ants or insects crawling on or under the skin.

Free radical: A highly reactive compound created by air pollution, radiation, cigarette smoke, or the incomplete breakdown of proteins and fats.

Gastritis: Inflammation of the stomach.

Gastrointestinal: Referring to the stomach and intestinal tract.

Glucose: A sugar; the building block of starch and glycogen.

Hemoglobin (a chelate): The iron-containing, oxygen-carrying protein in red blood cells.

High-density lipoprotein (HDL): A substance that includes fats and protein that transports fats in the blood away from the tissues. A high level of HDL is associated with a low risk for cardiovascular disease.

Hormone: A chemical substance produced by a group of cells or an organ (the endocrine glands) and circulating through the blood to regulate other organs. Examples are estrogen, adrenaline, and insulin.

Hydrogenated fat: An unsaturated fat such as a vegetable oil that has been processed with hydrogen to become more saturated. Margarine and shortening are examples.

Hyperglycemia: High blood sugar.

Hypertension: High blood pressure.

Hypoglycemia: Low blood sugar.

Hypotension: Low blood pressure.

Immune system: A complex system of body defenses that involves the hormones, cells, and tissues that protect the body from disease.

Insomnia: Chronic inability to sleep.

Irritable bowel syndrome (IBS): Also called spastic colon and mucous colitis. Chronic distention, rumbling, pain, diarrhea, or constipation not caused by identifiable organic disease.

Irritable syndrome: Irritability of any organ.

Lactose: A milk sugar.

Lactose intolerance. The inability to digest milk sugar due to low levels of lactase (an enzyme).

Linoleic acid: An essential polyunsaturated fatty acid of the Omega-6 family that cannot be produced by the body and must be supplied from dietary sources such as vegetable oils, especially warm-climate oils.

Linolenic acid: An essential polyunsaturated fatty acid of the Omega-3 family (see **Alpha linolenic**). This acid is found in cold-climate plants such as walnuts, soybeans, flaxseed, chestnuts, hazelnuts, winter wheat, and northern beans.

Lipids: Fats such as cholesterol and especially lecithin (a diglyceride).

Low density lipoprotein (LDL): A type of lipid-protein complex that tends to deposit fatty cholesterol in tissues and artery walls. A high level of LDL is dangerous.

Malignant: Having a life-threatening character. The term usually refers to cancerous conditions.

Ménière's syndrome: A disease of the

internal ear causing attacks of severe dizziness and other unpleasant symptoms such as nausea.

Metabolism: The sum of all body processes that convert foods into body tissues and energy. **Basal metabolism** is the minimum amount of energy required to maintain basic body processes.

Migraine headache: Intense pain in the head, often with changes in visual or other sensations and often confined to one side and accompanied by nausea and vomiting.

Monounsaturated: Fats with only one region of unsaturation, e.g., oleic acid, which is contained in olive oil in relatively high amounts.

Neurosis: Attacks of fear or other mental abberations not severe enough to cause loss of contact with reality.

Nitrite: A chemical compound that is added to processed meats as a preservative and coloring agent. It is converted in the stomach to the carcinogen nitrosamine.

Obesity: Body weight more than 20 percent above desirable weight; morbid overweight.

Omega: The last letter of the Greek alphabet; used by chemists to describe the last carbon atom in a chain.

Omega-3: A family of essential fatty acids of a very high polyunsaturated type in which unsaturation starts three carbons in from the end carbon.

Omega-6: A family of essential fatty acids of a very high polyunsaturated type in which unsaturation starts six carbons in from the end carbon.

Osteoporosis: Loss of calcium from the bone, resulting in reduced bone strength and increased fractures. The bone retains its diameter and length, but becomes less dense.

Ovary: The female endocrine gland located at the tip of the Fallopian tubes.

Pectin: A soluble nondigestible dietary fiber found in apples and many other fruits. Its consumption helps reduce elevated serum cholesterol.

Pellagra: A disease caused by deficiency of niacin (vitamin B_3). The symptoms are skin disorders (dermatitis), mental problems (dementia), diarrhea, weakness, and others.

Placebo: A medicine that has no specific chemical effect but may induce nonspecific psychological effects.

Platelet: One of the cells in the blood that aid in blood clotting.

Polyunsaturated fatty acid (PUFA): An unsaturated fat with two or more regions of unsaturation (double bonds) that is liquid at room temperature and is found in vegetable oils, nuts, seeds, and fish. Essentially similar to EFA.

Premenstrual tension syndrome (PMS): A combination of emotional and physical discomforts immediately prior to menstruation.

Pro-A (pro-vitamin A or **beta-carotene):** An essential nutrient converted in the body into vitamin A. Along with vitamins C and E and selenium, it is also an antioxidant and may act as an anticancer agent. Present in plant sources, especially leafy greens and yellow and red vegetables such as carrots, and egg yolk and milk fat. Commercial preparations from these sources are available as nutritional supplements that supply both pro-A and A. In contrast, pro-A is low or absent in the usual fish oil sources commonly used as nutritional supplements of vitamin A.

Prostaglandin (PG): A group of hormonelike substances formed from fatty acids and regulating body tissues in many ways. They stimulate or relax smooth muscles and blood vessels, among many other activities.

Prostate: A male sex gland, located just below the bladder and encircling the urethra at the point where it exits from the bladder. **Prostatitis** is prostate inflammation, which can cause frequency of urination. **Benign prostatic**

hypertrophy (BPH) causes similar problems.

Psychosis: A severe impairment of mental or emotional functions; an inability to evaluate reality correctly, often associated with hallucinations.

Recommended dietary allowances (RDA): The amounts of nutrients recommended by the Food and Nutrition Board of the National Academy of Sciences as the optimum required to meet the health needs of people in good health. The **minimum daily requirement (MDR)** is the minimum amount needed to maintain health.

Saturated fat: A type of fat that is solid at room temperature, often found in foods from animal sources and also in coconut and palm kernel oil. Unsaturated fats can be "saturated" by adding hydrogen during processing and preparation for distribution as food.

Schizophrenia: A psychosis mainly involving severe problems in organizing thoughts, with flattened emotion inappropriate to or split from thought context, often with hallucinations.

Scurvy: A bleeding disease caused by a deficiency of vitamin C.

Seborrheic dermatitis: Flaking and scaling of the skin between the nose and outer corners of the mouth or around the eyebrows or scalp, with reddening and irritation. It is often associated with scalp dandruff.

Stroke: A condition of impaired brain function resulting from hemorrhage or a blood clot of the vessels in the brain. It is the brain counterpart of a heart attack.

Substrate: A chemical compound that is converted into another compound via a chemical reaction. Also called a reactant.

Tinnitus: A ringing, swishing, or buzzing sound in the ears.

Trans-fatty acid: An abnormally shaped polyunsaturated fat found in very high concentrations in hydrogenated vegetable oils.

Type A personality: An aggressive, anxious, impatient, stressed person.

Tyramine: A metabolic product of amino acid.

Unsaturated fat: A fatty acid having reactive unsaturated regions or double bonds between carbon atoms where more hydrogen can be added.

Vaginal: Pertaining to the vagina.

Varicose veins: Enlarged or twisted veins that often appear in the legs.

Vein: One of the blood vessels that carry waste products from the tissues for eventual elimination.

Virus: Any of a large group of minute particles that are capable of infecting plants, animals, and humans.

Vitamin: An organic substance (often an "amine," hence *vit-amin*) essential to life and required in the diet by the body in very small amounts.

Xeroderma: Very dry skin.

Appendix A
Sources of Essential Fatty Acids

Food Omega Sources

The table on the following page lists the foods rich in Omega-3 and Omega-6 essential fatty acids (EFA) and gives their amounts as grams per 100 grams of food. To use the table, find the food of interest in the left column and read across to find the amount of EFA in 100 grams of that food. (NEFA indicates nonessential fatty acids.) The figures given have been compiled from a diversity of scientific sources. Values may vary with season, temperature, and nutrient source.

Food Sources of Essential Fatty Acids (EFA)

Compiled by J. M. Rudin

Sources	Grams per 100-gram portion				EFA	NEFA	Overall fat content	Cholesterol (mg. per 100 grams)
	Omega-6 EFA Linoleic	Omega-3 EFA Alpha-linolenic	EPA	DHA				
DAIRY PRODUCTS								
Butter	1.8	1.2			3.0	73	80	245
Cheeses: natural								
Cheddar	0.5	0.4			0.9	30	33	105
Cream	0.8	0.5			1.3	31	34	109
Gouda	0.3	0.4			0.7	25	27	112
Gruyère	1.3	0.4			1.7	29	32	109
Roquefort	0.7	0.8			1.5	31	34	75
Cheeses: Processed								
American	0.6	0.3			0.9	27	29	96
Cheddar	0.7	0.4			1.1	27	30	107
Cream, heavy	0.9	0.6			1.5	34	38	146
Cream, light	0.5	0.3			0.8	19	21	70
Cream, sour	0.4	0.3			0.7	17	18	45
Desserts								
Ice cream, vanilla	0.8	0.2			0.5	11	12	26
Pudding, tapioca	0.3	0.1			0.4	4	5	150
Milk, cow's	0.1	0.1			0.2	3	4	15
MILK, HUMAN								
Mature, W. Nigeria	2.3	0.09			2.4	13	15	
Mature, N. America	0.4	0.06	0.01	0.01	0.4	3	4	14
Mature, Australia	0.4	0.02			0.5	3	4	

EGGS								
Chicken, cooked in shell (1 large)	312	11	8	1.4			0.03	1.3
SEAFOOD								
Finfish, fillets								
Cod, Atlantic	50	0.7	0.21	0.26	0.15	0.08		0.01
Flounder	50	1.2	0.63	0.35	0.11	0.11	0.01	
Halibut, Atlantic	50	1.1	0.43	0.43	0.30	0.10	0.03	0.02
Halibut, Pacific	50	2.0	1.17	0.55	0.20	0.11	0.02	0.07
Halibut, Greenland	50	8.4	6.97	0.73	0.22	0.27	0.11	0.29
Herring, Atlantic	85	6.2	2.79	1.43	0.58	0.33	0.03	0.12
Herring, Pacific		11.1	8.50	1.67	0.57	0.76	0.10	0.14
Mackerel, Atlantic	95	9.8	6.70	2.44	1.10	0.65	0.23	0.43
Mackerel, Seer		15.5	11.60	2.63	1.30	0.49	0.02	0.04
Rockfish, canary	60	3.1	1.76	0.98	0.48	0.32	0.05	0.08
Salmon, Atlantic		5.8	4.74	0.51	0.13	0.18	0.11	0.13
Salmon, Chinook		13.2	9.59	2.49	0.72	1.00	0.04	0.08
Salmon, Coho, Pacific		7.5	4.57	2.28	0.94	0.82		
Salmon, Sockeye (canned)		6.7	2.66	3.44	1.00	0.62	0.41	0.15
Salmon, Sockeye	34	8.9	3.58	4.71	1.70	1.30	0.31	1.40
Sole, lemon		0.8	0.30	0.27	0.09	0.09		
Tuna, Albacore (canned)	50	6.8	4.30	1.81	1.10	0.38	0.04	0.05
Tuna, Bluefin (canned)	45	4.6	3.00	1.17	0.63	0.33	0.02	0.03
Shellfish								
Crab, Alaska King, legs & claws, cooked	100	1.6	0.70	0.62	0.15	0.33	0.04	0.03
Spiny lobster, flesh, Caribbean	200	1.2	0.20	0.59	0.09	0.18	0.01	0.03

Grams per 100-gram portion

Sources	Omega-6 EFA Linoleic	Omega-3 EFA Alpha-linolenic	EPA	DHA	EFA	NEFA	Overall fat content	Cholesterol (mg. per 100 grams)
Shrimp, different species, flesh	0.02	0.01	0.18	0.15	0.47	0.40	1.2	150
Clam, edible portion	0.03	0.02	0.08	0.07	0.28	0.45	1.4	120
Oyster, Pacific, flesh	0.03	0.04	0.42	0.29	0.90	0.58	2.3	50
Scallops, different species, flesh	0.01		0.12	0.14	0.35	0.2	0.91	35
Snail, pond, flesh	0.10	0.09		0.36	1.14	1.10	2.80	
FOWL (roasted)								
Chicken, dark meat	1.9	0.1		0.1	2.4	6.1	9.7	75
Chicken, light meat	1.3	0.1		0.1	1.6	4.0	6.4	53
Turkey, dark meat	1.1	0.1		0.2	1.5	3.1	5.3	98
Turkey, light meat	0.5	0.03		0.1	0.7	1.4	2.6	77
MEAT								
Beef (broiled)								
Steak, average of flank or sirloin	0.3	0.1			0.4	6.6	7.5	63
Ground, 77% lean	0.5	0.3			0.9	19.2	21.2	64
Lamb (roasted or broiled)								
Loin, 66% lean, 34% fat	1.2	0.6			1.9	28.7	32.4	60
Leg, 82% lean, 17% fat	0.8	0.3			1.2	18.2	21.2	70
Rib, 62% lean, 38% fat	1.4	0.7			2.1	32.0	36.0	70
Pork								
Ham (roasted or boiled), 84% lean, 16% fat	1.8	0.2			2.1	16.3	19.6	70

Spareribs (braised)	51	39.0	32.1	4.2	0.3	3.5
Bacon (smoked, cooked)	22	49.0	41.2	5.4	0.6	4.7
Lunch meat (canned)	70	30.1	25.0	3.6	0.4	3.1
Sausage, pork (cooked)	70	32.5	27.0	3.9	0.4	3.4
Sausages, pork & beef						
Bologna		27.5	24.1	2.1	0.3	1.7
Frankfurter		28.9	24.6	2.9	0.4	2.4
Vienna sausage		25.2	21.9	2.0	0.3	1.6
Veal loin (cooked, roasted), 85% lean, 15% fat	56	13.6	11.6	0.9	0.2	0.6
Organ meats						
Beef heart, lean cooked		0.7	3.3	1.1	0.01	0.7
Beef liver, lean (cooked)	150	10.6	9.1	1.5	0.1	1.1
Pork liver (cooked)	300	11.5	8.2	1.8	0.1	1.3
VEGETABLES—Omega-6 (tropical to temperate)						
Kernels, Nuts, & Seeds						
Cashews		46	36	7.5	0.2	7.3
Corn		50	19	29.0	0.5	28.5
Cottonseed		23	10	11.6	0.1	11.5
Olive		68	59	6.1	0.5	5.6
Peanut		50	32	15.0	0.6	14.4
Poppyseed		47	15	32.0		32.0
Pumpkin seed		33	15	17.0		17.0
Safflower		35	12	20.0		20.0
Sesame		48	27	19.2	0.2	19.2
Sunflower		27	15	12.0		12.0
Coconut		36	33	0.7	0.0	0.7

Grams per 100-gram portion

Sources	Omega-6 EFA Linoleic	Omega-3 EFA Alpha-linolenic	EPA	DHA	EFA	NEFA	Overall fat content	Cholesterol (mg. per 100 grams)
VEGETABLES—Omega-3 sources (temperate to polar)								
Kernels, nuts, & seeds								
Chestnut	17	20			19	40	50	
Linseed (flaxseed)	7	17			24	14	38	
Perilla	6	27			33	10	40	
Soybean	11	2			13	8	21	
Walnut, black	37	4			41	16	60	
Walnut, English	35	7			42	19	63	
Wheat germ	6	0.7			7	4	11	
Seeds, Leguminous								
Bean, common (kidney, navy, pinto, red)	0.3	0.6			0.9	0.3	1.5	
Broad bean	0.7	0.1			0.8	0.6	1.6	
Chickpea	2.2	0.1			2.3	1.6	5.0	
Cowpea	0.5	0.3			0.8	0.8	2.0	
Lentil	0.4	0.1			0.5	0.4	1.2	
Lima bean	0.4	0.2			0.7	0.4	1.4	
Garden pea, green (raw)	0.3	0.1			0.4	0.3	0.8	

NOTE: Almonds and hazelnuts have very little linolenic acid (Omega-3).

Food Oil Omega Sources

The table on the following page lists the food oils rich in Omega-3 and Omega-6 essential fatty acids (EFA) and gives their amounts in grams per 100 grams of food oil. To use the table, find the food oil of interest in the left column and read across to find the amount of EFA in 100 grams of that food oil. (NEFA indicates nonessential fatty acids.) The figures given have been compiled from a diversity of scientific sources. All oil data are for *non*hydrogenated oils. Values may vary with season, temperature, and nutrient source.

Food Oil Sources of Essential Fatty Acids (EFA)

Compiled by J. M. Rudin

Grams per 100-gram portion

Sources	Omega-6 EFA	Omega-3 EFA			EFA	NEFA	Overall fat content	Cholesterol (mg. per 100 grams)
	Linoleic	Alpha linolenic	EPA	DHA				
FISH OILS								
Cod, Atlantic	1.2	0.8	12.4	21.9	41.7	57.7	100	
Halibut, Pacific	0.9	0.3	10.1	7.9	26.9	72.0	100	
Mackerel	1.1	1.3	7.1	10.8	29.3	71.0	100	
Rockfish	1.6	0.8	11.7	17.4	36.1	63.0	100	
Salmon, Chinook	1.1	0.9	8.2	5.9	20.6	80.0	100	
Salmon, Coho	1.2	0.6	12.0	13.8	33.6	65.2	100	
Sole, lemon	0.7	2.0	14.7	6.8	36.6	58.0	100	
Tuna, albacore	0.7	0.6	6.5	17.6	29.6	69.0	100	
Tuna, bluefin	1.3	tr.	6.6	20.8	33.5	66.6	100	
FISH LIVER OIL								
Cod, Atlantic (toxic at high doses)	1.5	0.9	8.0	14.3	29.7	68.0	100	1000
SHELLFISH OILS								
Oyster, Pacific	1.2	1.6	21.5	20.2	51.7	48.2	100	
Scallops, sea	0.6	0.3	21.3	26.2	55.7	44.3	100	
VEGETABLE OILS—								
Omega-6 sources (tropical to temperate)								
Cashew	16	0.4			16	79	100	
Corn	57	0.8			58	37	100	

Cottonseed	48	0.4	48	49	100	
Evening primrose*	72	0.2	81	20	100	0.1
Olive	9	0.7	10	89	100	
Peanut	29	1.1	30	68	100	
Poppyseed	69		69	31	100	
Pumpkin seed	51		51	45	100	
Safflower	58		58	33	100	
Sesame	42		42	56	100	
Sunflower	53		46	55	100	
Coconut oil	3	0.5	3	96	100	
VEGETABLE OILS—						
Omega-3 sources						
(temperate to polar)						
Chestnuts, European	35	4	3.9	50	100	
Hempseed	62	19	81	21	100	
Linseed	18	45	63	36	100	
Perilla	16	67	83	26	100	
Soybean	53	7	60	39	100	
Walnut	67	4	71	21	100	
Walnut, black	62	7	69	27	100	
Walnut, English	55	11	66	29	100	
Wheat germ	54	7	61	33	100	
ANIMAL FATS						
Beef tallow	4	0.7	4.2	92	100	
Chicken fat	17	1.1	17.6	78	100	
Lard	10	1.4	11.8	84	100	
Mutton fat	5	2.9	8.1	88	100	

*Contains 8.6 grams of gamma linolenic.

Appendix B
For Those Who Want
More Information

REFERENCES

GENERAL REFORM NUTRITION

Berland, T. *Consumer Guide's Rating the Diets.* New York: New American Library, 1979.

Burkitt, D. *Eat Right—To Keep Healthy and Enjoy Life More.* New York: Arco, 1979.

Century 21 Cookbook: 375 Meatless Recipes. Leominster, Mass.: The Eusey Press, Inc., 1974.

Chapman, N. T. *Bean Cuisine.* Toronto: Rebecca Clarkes Pub., 1984.

Cheraskin, E., *et al. Lower Your Cholesterol in 30 Days.* New York: Putnam, 1986.

Childers, N. F., *Childers' Diet to Stop Arthritis.* Somerset Press, 1981.

Cleave, T. L. *The Saccharine Disease: The Master Disease of Our Time.* New Canaan, CT: Keats, 1975.

Colbin, A. *The Book of Whole Meals.* Brookline, Mass.: Autumn Press, 1979.

Collier, C. *The Natural Sugarless Dessert Cookbook.* New York: Walker and Co., 1980.

Crook, W. G. *The Yeast Connection,* 3rd edition. Jackson, TN.: Prof. Books, 1986.

Davis, Adelle. *Let's Get Well.* New York: New American Library, 1965.

Ellis, J. M., and Presley, J. *Vitamin B_6: The Doctor's Report.* New York: Harper and Row, 1973.

Elrick, H., Crakes, H., and Clarke, S. *Living Longer and Better.* New York: World Publications, 1978.

Ewald, E. B. *Recipes for a Small Planet.* New York: Ballantine, 1973.

Fredericks, C. *Eat Well, Get Well, Stay Well.* New York: Grosset and Dunlap, 1980.

Gibbons, B. *The Slim Gourmet Cookbook.* New York: Harper and Row, 1976.

———. *The Year-Round Turkey Cookbook.* New York: McGraw-Hill, 1980.

Guerard, M. *Michel Guerard's Cuisine Minceur.* New York: Bantam, 1976.

Harris, W. S., *et al.* "Dietary Omega-3 Fatty Acids Prevent Carbohydrate Induced Hypertriglyceridemia." *Metabolism* 33:1016–19, 1984.

Hausman, P. *Calcium Bible.* New York: Rawson Associates, 1985.

Hoffer, A., and Osmond, H. *How to Live with Schizophrenia.* Secaucus, NJ: Citadel Press, 1978.

Hoffer, A., and Walker, M. *Orthomolecular Nutrition.* New Canaan, CT: Keats, 1978.

Hoffer, R., and Warrington, M. *Everybody's Favorite Orthomolecular Muffin Book.* New, Canaan, CT: Keats, 1980.

Horrobin, D. F. *Clinical Uses for Essential Fatty Acids.* St. Albans, VT: Eden Press, 1983.

Kane, P. *Food Makes the Difference.* New York: Simon and Schuster, 1985.

Kloss, J. *Back to Eden.* Santa Barbara, CA: Woodbridge, 1975.

Kremer, J. M., *et al.* "Effects of Manipulation of Dietary Fatty Acids on Clinical Manifestations of Rheumatoid Arthritis. *Lancet* 1:184–7, 1985.

Kromhaut, D., *et al.* "Inverse Relation Between Fish Consumption and 20 year Mortality from Coronary Heart Disease. *New England Journal of Medicine* 312:1205–9, 1985.

Kunin, R. A. *Meganutrition: The New Prescription for Maximum Health, Energy and Longevity.* New York: New American Library, 1981.

Kushi, M. *The Book of Macrobiotics.* Japan Publications, Inc. 1977.

Lappe, F. M. *Diet for a Small Planet.* New York: Ballantine, 1975.

Mandell, M., and Scanlon, L. W. *Dr. Mandell's Five Day Allergy Relief System.* New York: Crowell, 1979.

Nidetch, J., *Weight Watchers Food Plan Diet Cookbook.* New York: New American Library, 1982.

Pauling, L. *How to Live Longer and Feel Better.* New York: Freeman, 1986.

Pfeiffer, C. C. *Mental and Elemental Nutrients.* New Canaan, CT: Keats, 1975.

Polunin, M. *The Wholegrain Health-Saver Book.* New Canaan, CT: Keats, 1982.

Reuben, D. *The Save Your Life Diet.* New York: Ballantine, 1976.

Reuben, D., and Reuben, B. *The Save Your Life Diet High Fiber Cookbook.* New York: Ballantine, 1977.

Rimland, B. *Infantile Autism.* Englewood Cliffs, NJ: Prentice-Hall, 1964.

Robertson, L., *et al. Laurel's Kitchen: A Handbook for Vegetarian Cookery and Nutrition.* New York: Bantam, 1976.

Rombauer, I. S., and Becker, M. R. *Joy of Cooking.* New York: Bobbs-Merrill, 1964.

Seelig, M. *Magnesium Deficiency in the Pathogenesis of Disease.* New York: Plenum, 1980.

Tarnower, H., and Baker, S. S. *The Complete Scarsdale Diet.* New York: Bantam, 1978.

Trowell, H. C., and Burkitt, D. P. *Western Diseases: Their Emergence and Prevention.* Cambridge, MA: Harvard University Press, 1981.

Trowell, H., Burkitt, D., and Heaton, D. (eds). *Dietary Fibre, Fibre-Depleted Foods and Disease.* New York: Academic Press, 1985.

Walford, R. L. *Maximum Lifespan.* New York: W. W. Norton, 1983.

White, B. *Bean Cuisine.* Boston: Beacon Press, 1977.

Wright, J. V. *Dr. Wright's Guide to Healing with Nutrition.* Emmaus, Pa.: Rodale, 1984.

ALLERGY

Merck Manual. "Elimination Diets," Table 18-1, p. 308, 14th ed. Merck Sharp and Dohme Research Laboratories, 1982.

Merck Manual. "Gluten Free Diet," Table 11-20, p. 1143, 13 ed. Merck, Sharp and Dohme Research Laboratories, 1977.

Rawcliffe, P. *The Glutein-Free Diet Book.* New York: Arco, 1985.

Stevens, L. J. *The Complete Book of Allergy Control.* New York: Macmillan, 1983.

U.S. Air Force. *Gluten Restricted Diet,* 1983.

EXERCISE

Bowerman, W. J., and Harris, W. E. *Jogging.* New York: Grosset and Dunlap, 1967.

Fixx, J. F. *The Complete Book of Running.* New York: Random House, 1977.

Morehouse, L. E. *Total Fitness in 30 Minutes a Week.* New York: Simon and Schuster, 1975.

Runner's World Editors. *New Exercises for Runners.* Cleveland: World Publications, 1978.

Sheehan, G. A. *Dr. Sheehan on Running.* Cleveland: World Publications, 1975.

Southmayd, W., and Hoffman, M. *Sports Health: The Complete Book of Athletic Injuries.* New York: Quick Fox, 1981.

STRESS RELIEF

Benson, H. *The Relaxation Response.* New York: William Morrow, 1975.

Hoffer, A., and Osmond, H. *How to Live with Schizophrenia.* Secaucus, NJ: Citadel Press, 1978.

Iyengar, B. K. S. *Light on Yoga.* New York: Schocken Books, 1979.

Rogers, C. R. *Client Centered Therapy.* Boston: Houghton-Mifflin, 1951.

Schauss, A. G. *Diet, Crime and Delinquency.* Berkeley, CA: Parker House, 1981.

Selye, H. *Stress in Health and Disease.* Stoneham, MA: Butterworth, 1976.

MEDICAL MATTERS

Beasely, J. D. *The Impact of Nutrition on the Health of Americans. Report to the Ford Foundation, 1981.* Boston: Little Brown, 1983.

Bollet, A. J. "The Conquest of Pellagra." *Medical Times,* pp. 19–28, Nov. 1982.

Dukes, M. N. *Side Effects of Drugs.* New York: Elsevier, 1984.

Goodhart, R. S., and Shils, M. E. *Modern Nutrition in Health and Disease.* Philadelphia: Lea and Febiger, 1980 (pp. 1007–18).

Hayes, K. C., and Hegsted, D. M. "Toxicity of the Vitamins." In: *Toxicants Occurring Naturally in Foods* (pp. 235–53). Nat'l. Acad. Sci., 1973.

Horrobin, D. *The Prostaglandins.* St. Albans, VT: Eden Press, 1978.

Merck Manual, 14th ed. "Nutrition: General Considerations—List of Nutrient Uses and Toxicities." pp. 870–7. Rahway, NJ: Merck, Sharp and Dohme Research Laboratories, 1982.

Merck Manual of Diagnosis and Therapy, 14th ed. Rahway, NJ: Merck, Sharp and Dohme Research Laboratories, 1982.

NAS/NRC. *Recommended Dietary Allowances,* 9th ed, 1980.

Physician's Desk Reference, 39th ed. Oradell, NJ: Medical Economics, 1985.

NUTRITION PUBLICATIONS OF DONALD O. RUDIN, M.D.

"The Major Psychoses and Neuroses as Omega-3 Essential Fatty Acid Deficiency Syndrome: Substrate Pellagra." *Biol. Psychiat.* 16:837–49, 1981.

"The Dominant Diseases of Modernized Societies as Omega-3 Essential Fatty Acid Deficiency Syndrome: Substrate Beriberi." *Medical Hypotheses* 8:17–47, 1982.

"The Three Pellagras." *J. Orthomol. Psychiat.* 12(2):91–110, 1983.

"Pellagra Extended." *Newsletter Soc. for Environ. Therapy,* 3(2):3–7, 1983.

"The Doctor's Forum" (On Aging and Nutrition). In: *Your Good Health,* 1(8):38–39, Dec. 1983.

"Time for a Primary Health Care Profession: Call for a National Conference to Form the American Federation of Primary Health Care Societies." *Int. J. Biosocial Res.* 5:55–56, 1983; also *J. Orthmol. Psychiat.* 13(1):25–26, 1984.

"On Essential Fatty Acids: An Interview." In: *Health News and Review.* July–August 1984 (p. 4).

"Omega-3 Essential Fatty Acids in Medicine." In: *1984–85 Yearbook of Nutritional Medicine,* Bland, J. (ed.). New Canaan, CT: Keats, 1985 (pp. 37–54).

"Omega-3 Essential Fatty Acid Deficiency as a Central Component of a Synergistic Malnutrition Causing the Modernization Diseases: Lipid Substrate Pellagra-Beriberi as a New Diagnostic Entity." *Proc. Br. Soc. for Nutritional Medicine Meeting on EFA,* October, 1985, England (in press, 1987).

"The Modernization Disease Syndrome as Substrate Pellagra-Berberi: A New Diagnostic Entity: Synergistic Malnutrition from Interacting Food Modifications." *J. Orthomol. Medicine* 2(1), pp. 3–14 (1987).

LECTURE TAPES by Donald O. Rudin

"The Nutritional Missing Link and the Modernization Diseases": Huxley Conference, 1981 (Boston), 1983 (New Orleans).
American Schizophrenia Association: Huxley Institute for Biosocial Research
900 North Federal Highway, Suite 330
Boca Raton, FL 33432
(305) 393-6167

"Essential Fatty Acids in Human Health and Disease": AIMS Fox Hollow Symposium, Dec. 3–5, 1982. Set of 11 Audiocassettes.
Creative Audio
87551 Osborne
Highland, IN 46322
(219) 838-2770

"Omega Disease: The New Pellagra": Canadian Schizophrenia Foundation, April 15, 1985, Toronto, Canada.
Kennedy Recordings
RR#5
Edmonton, Alberta T5P 4B7
Canada

NUTRITION NEWSPAPERS AND NEWSLETTERS

Bio-Nutrionics Newsletter
Dept 62B, Bio-Nutrionics
120 E. 56th St.
New York, NY 10022

Better Nutrition
Syndicate Magazines, Inc.
6 E. 43d St.
New York, NY 10017

Executive Health
Executive Health Publications
P.O. Box 589
Rancho Santa Fe, CA 92067

*The Felix Letter: A Commentary on
  Nutrition*
P.O. Box 7094
Berkeley, CA 94707

For You, Naturally
Tele-Health
R.D. #3, Clymer Rd.
Quakertown, PA 18951

Health News and Review,
Johlian Publishing Co., Inc.
670 Merrick Rd.
Lynbrook, NY 11563

Natural Health Bulletin
Parker Publishing Co.
Rt. 59A at Brookhill Drive
West Nyack, NY 10994

Nutrition Action
Center for Science in the Public
  Interest
1501 16th St. N.W.
Washington, D.C. 20036

Nutrition and the M.D.
PM Inc.
6931 Van Nuys Blvd.
P.O. Box 2160
Van Nuys, CA 91405

Nutrition Health Review
171 Madison Ave.
New York, NY 10016

Nutrition Today
Nutrition Today, Inc.
703 Giddings Ave.
Annapolis, MD 21404

Nutritional Update
Keats Publishing Co.
36 Grove St.
New Canaan, CT 06840

*Newsletter for the Society of
  Environmental Therapy*
31 Sarah St.
Darwen, Lancashire BB3 3ET
England

Professional Nutritionist
2226 Clay St.
San Francisco, CA 94115

R. P. Scherer Survey of Health and
  Nutrition Literature
P.O. Box 7220
Silver Spring, MD 20907

*Woman's Day—Today's Woman's Diet
  and Exercise Guide*
CBS Publications
1515 Broadway
New York, NY 10036

Your Good Health, Review and Digest
Keats Publishing Co.
27 Pine St., P.O. Box 876
New Canaan, CT 06840

CONTACTS TO FIND THE NAMES OF PRACTICING REFORM NUTRITIONISTS AND PHYSICIANS

American Holistic Medical Association
6932 Little River Turnpike
Annandale, VA 22003
(703) 642-5880

Bio-Nutrionics
Dept. 62 B
120 E. 56th St.,
New York, NY 10022
1-800-STAMINA

Canadian Schizophrenia Foundation
2229 Broad St.
Regina, Saskatchewan S4P 1Y7
Canada
(306) 757-7969

Huxley Institute for Biosocial Research
American Schizophrenia Association
900 N. Federal Highway, Suite 330
Boca Raton, FL 33432
(305) 393-6167

Northwest Academy of Preventive Medicine
15615 Bellevue-Redmond Road, Suite E
Bellevue, WA 98008
(206) 881-9660

TO FIND A RELIABLE M.D.

Call your local medical society or, if the problem seems to be serious, call the office of the head of the Department of Medicine or appropriate specialty of your nearest medical school or medical school–affiliated hospital.

Appendix C
The Modernization Disease Syndrome as Substrate Pellagra-Beriberi

A New Diagnostic Entity: Synergistic Malnutrition from Interacting Food Modifications

Donald O. Rudin, M.D.

A scientific article on the general biomedical significance of Omega-3 EFA and nutrition for the modernization disease syndrome

Reprinted by permission from the *Journal of Orthomolecular Medicine* 2(1), pp. 3–14, 1987.

ABSTRACT

Today's multiple food manipulations may interact to produce a widespread difficult-to-identify *synergistic malnutrition* presenting as a highly idiosyncratic substrate-catalyst-antinutrient vitamin-resistant Hoffer-type pellagra-beriberi mainly afflicting primates and accounting for the medically dominant modernization disease *syndrome* as a variant of the classical catalytic B vitamin-sensitive Goldberger-Eijkman-Takaki pellagra-beriberi.

Key words: *beriberi, essential fatty acid, pellagra, malnutrition, modernization disease.*

INTRODUCTION

Authorities now link distortions of dietary fats to both the number 1 and 2 killers, namely, heart disease and certain major cancers, especially breast, prostate, and colon (1,2). But saturated and polyunsaturated essential fatty acids (EFA) have also long been implicated, *particularly in primates,* in arthritis (3), immune diseases (4–8), diabetes (9–13), eczemas (14), polyneuropathies (15), behavioral disorders including schizophrenia (16–21), cystic fibrosis (19), and other problems ranging from drying skin disorders to irritable bowel syndrome (20,21).

Most of these newly prominent illnesses do not seem to result from diagnostic or therapeutic advances, for many are diagnostically striking, occur in the young or middle aged, have been tracked by medical officers as societies modernize, e.g., hypertension and schizophrenia (18,22) across the South Sea islands. The conservative assumption is that they may constitute a highly idiosyncratic modernization diseases syndrome (MDS) in response to multiple interacting food manipulations adversely affecting co- and antinutrients which interact synergistically in the body to disrupt the body-wide lipid-based regulatory system, including prostaglandins, in ways depending on genetic susceptibility.

Abbreviations: Linoleic acid, LA = 18.2ω6; γ-linolenic acid, GLA = 18:3ω6; dihomogamma-linolenic acid, DGLA = 20:3ω6; arachidonic acid, AA = 20:4ω6; α-linolenic acid, ALA = 18:3ω3; eicosapentaenoic acid, EPA = 20:5ω3; docosahexaenoic acid, DHA = 22:6ω3. The italic numbers in parentheses refer to the numbered references given at the end of this article.

THE REACTION COHERENCE OF ESSENTIAL NUTRIENTS

Most of the approximately fifty essential nutrients comprise a set of coreactants: (1) substrates, including lipids, (2) B-vitamin containing enzymes which process the lipids into products comprising the lipid regulatory system including prostaglandins and steroid derivatives, and (3) modulators, such as the EFA-protecting antioxidants (vitamins A, C, and E and selenium) as well as dietary fiber, which acts as the prime regulator of fat metabolism in the gut, thus, indirectly determining systemic EFA requirements. In addition, various dietary antinutrients, such as saturated fat, cholesterol, and sugar, interfere with these conutrients in the *Fundamental Reaction of Nutrition:*

EAA (10) ──────────┐   ┌───► Structural and regulatory proteins

              __B vitamin enzymes__

              co- & anti-modulators

EFA($\omega 6/\omega 3$) ◄────┘   └───► Structural and regulatory lipids:
                                                   (PG 1,2/3,4; chol- & glyc-EFA esters)

Since the co- and antinutrients form a coherent reaction schema, there can be four limiting pellagra-beriberiform disease variants, namely, substrate, catalyst cofactor, modulator, antinutrient and their combinations, e.g., vitamin B deficiency schizophrenia, irritable bowel syndrome, arthritis, etc.; EFA substrate deficiency schizophrenia, irritable bowel syndrome, etc., modulator schizophrenia, etc.; antinutrient schizophrenia, etc.; and the combined forms. Because the lipid products constitute a body-wide local tissue regulatory system—the tophormones—gene-dependent variations will produce a complex idiosyncratic or statistical illness structure—MDS will be identifiable not by examining the "patient as a whole" but only by a statistical or *epidemiological diagnosis.*

EVIDENCE FOR DIETARY DEVIATIONS FROM THE TRADITIONAL STANDARD

Evidence for significant systematic damage to the modern diet is presented, first, in Table 1, which gives the nutrient values of a prototypical neomodern daily diet (post 1965, with relatively high $\omega 6$ intake) compared with the same diet in its traditional *indigenous* and unprocessed form, corrected for changes in national dietary patterns over the past 100 years (e.g., 250% increase in sugar consumption) to approximate the prototypical temperate and cold-climate diet of 1850 or earlier.

The table shows that dietary availability of the more fluid cold-climate $\omega 3$-EFA in the neomodern diet is only 20% of the traditional diet (mainly as the result of increased consumption of $\omega 3$ deficient warm-climate oils, hydrogenation, decreased fish consumption and loss of cereal germ by machine milling) while more viscous warm-climate $\omega 6$ availability has changed little. Severe dietary fiber deficiency of about 75% exists, confirming findings of the British fiber theorists (*22*). Selenium intake is low, of interest since veterinarians find that livestock suffers from a widespread selenium deficiency of uncertain origin (*21*). Sugar consumption has risen 250%. Fatty acid *isomer* consumption has soared 2500% (hydrogenation) and from data on competitive enzyme inhibition (*23*) and isomer consumption levels, I calculate that 20–40% of EFA metabolic enzyme activity is blocked in the average person in the U.S., even as we reduce $\omega 3$-EFA availability by 80% and adversely affect its processing through conutrient deficiencies of fiber, selenium, and B vitamins as well as interfering antinutrient increases. The intake of cholesterol, saturated fat, and B vitamins varies widely, but the first two are significantly increased while vitamin B consumption may be reduced as much as 50% below the RDA in 20% of the population, mainly those consuming high levels of sugar (*24*).

Studies show that most of these nutritional deviations interfere synergistically with EFA utilization (*25*), thus effectively increasing EFA requirement, even as $\omega 3$-EFA availability declines. Consequently, the *effective* $\omega 3$-EFA equivalent deficiency is greatly in excess of the 80% dietary depletion. Evidence also indicates that lack of exercise in the face of an atherogenic diet in primates contributes significantly to atherosclerosis (*26*). In addition, the work of Selye (*27*) and others shows that stress also acts through the EFA-steroid system.

TABLE I
Food Damage Report for 1983:
Ancestral and Neo-Modern Diets Compared For Fatty Acids
and Other Components

Calories	Serving (grams)	Ancestral Food	ω3-EFA (gm)	ω6-EFA (gm)	NEFA (gm)	NeoModern Food	ω3-EFA (gm)	ω6-EFA (gm)	NEFA (gm)
600	3 cups (200)	Stone gnd wheat	0.2	2.5	2.0	1.5 cups refnd wheat	0.0	0.0	0.0
250	3 serv.	Fruit/grns	0.0	0.0	0.0	Fruit/grns	0.0	0.0	0.0
80	1 serv.	1 egg	0.0	1.3	8.0	1 egg	0.0	1.3	8.0
100	1 tblsp (15)	Butter	0.2	0.7	14.0	Margarine	0.2	4.0	11.0
100	1 serv. (80)	Tunafish	1.1	0.1	2.7	Hamburger (60 gm)	0.2	0.4	14.0
200	1 serv. (80)	Pork/Chick. (?hyd. feed)	0.2	2.0	20.0	Beefsteak (100) gm	0.4	0.8	26.0
150	1 cup (115)	Common bean (navy, kid.)	0.6	0.3	0.3	Asparagus (etc.)	0.0	0.0	0.0
150	¼ cup (35)	Walnuts (English)	1.5	9.0	5.0	Peanuts (Cashews)	0.1	3.0	8.0
150	2 tblsp (30)	Honey	0.0	0.0	0.0	Sugar 4tb (60 gm)	0.0	0.0	0.0
220	2 tblsp (30)	Soybean oil (Lard)	2.0 (0.4)	16.0 (3.5)	12.0 (25.0)	Cottonseed (hyd. soy)	0.1 (0.7)	15.0 (11.4)	15.0 (18.0)
2000			5.8	31.9	64.0		1.0	24.5	82.0

	Ancestral		NeoModern	
Total Fat	101.7 gm	= 43% of cal.	107.5 gm	= 46% of cal.
ω3-EFA	5.8 gm	= 2.5% of cal. (5.7% of oil)	1.0 gm	= 0.4% of cal. (1.0% of oil)
ω6-EFA	31.9 gm	= 14% of cal. (31% of oil)	24.5 gm	= 10% of cal. (23% of oil)
ω3/ω6	0.2		0.04	
Total EFA	37.7 gm		25.5 gm	
Isomer Index	0.4% of EFA		10.0% of EFA (hyd. soy)	
Vitamin E	60.0 mg		50.0 mg	
Selenium	260.0 mcg		75.0 mcg	
NEFA	64.0 gm		82.0 gm	
Sat. Fat	25.0 gm		34.0 gm	
Cholest.	480.0 mg		520.0 mg	
B vitamins	high		variable, low	
Fiber	25.0 gm		8.0 gm	
Salt	2.0 gm		10.0 gm	

Table I. Prototypical modern diet on the right and its unadulterated traditional equivalent on the left compared for all food values emphasizing EFA.

Refs: **EFA & Isomers:** Exler, J., et al., J. Am. Dietetic Assoc. 71:518, 1977; Carpenter, D. L., et al., JAOCS 53:713, 1976; Smith, L. M., et al., JAOC 55:257, 1978; Kirschman, J. D., Nutr. Almanac. McGraw-Hill, 1979. **Salt:** Goodhart, R. S., and Shils, M. E., Mod. Nutr. in Health and Disease, Lea & Febiger, 1973 (1011-14). **Statistics:** Historical Statistics, U.S. Consumer expendit. patterns, 1949-1970, (829-31); Ann. Rpt. Nut. Fd. Survey Comm., Household Food Consumption, 1973, Gov't Stationery Office, London.

DIETARY DEVIATIONS AND DISEASE CORRELATIONS

The results of Table 1 are supported by analyses of national dietary consumption patterns and related studies shown in Table 2, which compare ω3 and ω6-EFA consumption in individuals, animal colonies, and nations having a relatively low incidence of modernization diseases with others having reduced ω3-EFA consumption and a high incidence of heart disease, schizophrenia, arthritis, phrynoderma, polyneuropathies, Meniere's disease, and other illnesses (see Table 2 references).

The general results of Table 2 also indicate that the intake of ω3-EFA has been reduced about 80% in the unhealthy state compared to the healthy state while ω6 consumption is unchanged. Therefore, the Table 1 data are entered into Table 2 as Study #1.

Study #2 of Table 2 compared the ω3 and ω6-EFA consumption in German-occupied Norway. During this two-year period the incidence of cancer, heart disease, and schizophrenia all plummeted by a remarkable 40–50% and then rose again shortly afterwards, data collection being constant according to the authors of these studies. During this time, when the health improved, ω6-EFA consumption was again unchanged while ω3 consumption increased fivefold. However, there was also a general reversion to indigenous unprocessed food during the occupation, implying that other dietary cofactors such as fiber, sugar, and beef intake also normalized (see Table 1 and below).

Study #3 compared the EFA consumption in controls and children having phrynoderma (literally, "frog skin") in *warm-climate* India, where the differential requirement for ω3 relative to ω6-EFA is probably considerably less. In this case, which involved near starvation, there was a limitation on EFA intake of both types among the ill children while the healthy children consumed about twice as much of both families. The phrynoderma cleared over four to six months on linseed oil and other polyunsaturate supplements.

Study #4 gives the EFA consumption of Japanese in Japan versus the United States around 1960, before there was as much modernization of the diet in Japan as today. The incidence of bowel cancer and heart disease was found to be much higher in Japanese Americans and equaled that of U.S. citizens generally (*1,2*). The ω6-EFA consumption was, again, about the same in the two Japanese groups but the ω3 consumption of Japanese Americans was only 20% of the consumption in Japan. Meniere's and other diseases increasing in Japan following World War II are associated by Japanese investigators with increased fat consumption as dietary habits Westernize (*20,21*).

Study #5 compared the EFA consumption of Eskimos and Danes, the former having a much lower incidence of heart disease and osteoarthritis and about twice the Omega-3 EFA intake. However, as a cross-racial study, interpretive caution is necessary.

Study #6 suggested that Omega-3 EFA consumption in Britain is low and recommended supplementation with fish oils.

Study #7 examined a child with an abdominal gunshot wound placed on total parenteral nutrition using low ω3-EFA containing safflower oil (<0.5% ω3, 60% ω6) as sole EFA source. Over 4 months she developed a variety of severe neuropathies which were rapidly corrected by substituting high ω3-EFA containing soybean oil (10% ω3, 60% ω6) for the safflower oil. EFA serum profile studies established that her *acute* illnesses were the *specific* result of an ω3-EFA deficiency which was *specifically* cured by ω3-EFA supplementation with *non-hydrogenated* soybean oil.

Study #8 raised a colony of six Capuchins from infancy on a standard laboratory diet which would be regarded as healthy by all modern nutritionists using corn oil as sole EFA source (0.5% ω3, 60% ω6). By age two, all the animals developed (1) drying and scaling Dermatitis and alopecia, (2) two developed intractable Diarrhea and (3) developed a vicious genital self-mutilating Dementia, which would be called the "van Gogh" syndrome in psychiatry, where it is seen in both schizophrenia and mental retardation. While no single animal in this study showed all three of the classical three D's of pellagra, namely, Dermatitis, Diarrhea, and Dementia, *the colony as a whole did*. This shows the importance of making what may be called a statistical, epidemiological or demographic diagnosis, which goes entirely beyond the medical adage to "study the patient as a whole," since a true idiosyncratic illness can only be diagnosed by *studying the group as a whole*. In fact, the diagnosis was missed even by the authors of this study. Except for the self-mutilators, which were put out of their misery, all the animals recovered within *a few months* on adding linseed oil supplements (60% ω3, 20% ω6).

TABLE 2
Estimated Average MDRs and RDAs for the EFA

Study	ω3-EFA "Healthy" (% cal)	ω3-EFA "Unhealthy" (% cal)	ω6-EFA§ "Healthy" (% cal)	ω6-EFA§ "Unhealthy" (% cal)
1. Traditional vs Neo-modern Diet (1) (Table 1)	2%	0.4%	14%	10%
2. Norwegian Food Survey (2) (peacetime vs wartime)	>1%	0.4%	8%	5%
Norwegian Linseed Study (3)	2%	0.4%	8%	5%
3. Children-India (Healthy (vs phrynoderma) (4)	1%	0.5%	2%	1%
4. Jap./Am. Food Survey (5)	2%*	0.4%	6%	6%
5. Eskimo/Dane Food Survey (6)	2%*	1.0%	2%	5%
6. British Food survey (7)	<1.0%	<7%		
7. Parenteral child (8)	0.6%**	0.1%	4%	6%
8. Capuchin Study (Linseed oil vs corn oil) (9)	2%	0.2%	10%	15%
9. Rat Study (Brain func) (Soy vs safflower oil) (10)	1–2%	0.1%	10%	10%

Therefore: MDR (ω3-EFA) = 1% of calories; RDA (ω3-EFA) = 2% of calories
         MDR (ω6-EFA) = 2–3% of calories; RDA (ω6-EFA) = 5–10% of calories

Table 2. Various studies making estimates of national or individual consumption of Omega-3 and Omega-6 EFA for the healthy vs the unhealthy state.
§These are upper limits, since ω6 may be lost as isomers on hydrogenation.
*Japanese and Eskimo maritime diets are high in 5ω3 and 6ω3, which are, in some ways, more potent than 3ω3. Japanese were assumed to take 20% of calories as fat, otherwise 40% was assumed in all calculations when authors did not provide % of calories.
**This is a parenteral value and does not allow for losses in the gut or intake of normal nutrients, which probably increase EFA requirement.

Study #9 raised rats *over a full life cycle* on soybean oil as sole EFA source (10% ω3, 60% ω6). As adults, they showed significantly better maze performance than did lifetime controls on safflower oil (<0.5% ω3, 60% ω6). Compared with the prominent, even catastrophic, illnesses and their relatively rapid development in the primates in Study #8, this longterm result in rats plus other evidence (21) suggests that primates have a much greater dependence on ω3-EFA than do subprimates. In fact, ω3 EFA can be the dominant EFA in brain. (RDA ω3 and ω6-EFA in temperate climates is about 1–2% and 6–8% of calories.)

MALNUTRITIONAL SYNERGY

These findings suggest that a widespread fat-centered substrate and mixed pellagra-beriberiform disease resulting from a synergistic malnutrition could account for the modernization diseases. According to the Fundamental Reaction of Nutrition, we can form a synergistic malnutritional index:

The synergistic malnutritional index, $I_{sm} = (1 + \Sigma b_j y_j)/\pi(1 - a_i)\hat{x}_i =$ optimize; where $\hat{x}_i$ and y_j, i, j = 1,2,3, . . . , are the set of co- and antinutrient intake levels, respectively, and the $0 < a_i < 1$ and $b_j > 1$ are their respective synergy *vectors*.

For example, evidence indicates that Omega-3 EFA, dietary fiber, and niacin supplements independently lower serum fats (28–30) while both human and animal studies (31) show that skin and musculoskeletal disorders can be ameliorated by supplements of either EFA or B vitamins, the best results being obtained from combined synergistic therapy.

Omega-3 EFA also suppress tumorogenesis in lower animals while Omega-6 EFA seem to be required for carcinogenic transformation. Dietary linseed oil supplements dramatically reduce the incidence of liver tumors in rats given oral carcinogens while marine dietary oil supplements suppress mammary tumorogenesis in rats *(32)*. Other studies *(33)* suggest that mammary tumor enhancement is more likely to be related to Omega-6 prostaglandins than Omega-3 and may even require Omega-6 EFA. At the same time, mammary tumor suppression is reported with dietary supplements of the EFA-preserving antioxidants, vitamin E and selenium *(34)*. Conversely, tumor enhancement occurs with selenium deficiency *(35)* while both selenium and EFA supplements enhance inmmunocompetence *(36,37)*. Just as fats uncovered by antioxidants enhance mammary tumorogenesis, so fats uncovered by fiber enhance colon cancer *(38)*. Of course, ω3-EFA are also now held to be important in normalizing cardiovascular physiology *(1)*.

These findings suggest a resolution to the conflicting recommendation for increasing and decreasing polyunsaturate consumption by the Heart *(1)* and Cancer *(2)* Panels, respectively. By increasing ω-3 EFA and decreasing ω-6 EFA consumption, the public can at once lower total polyunsaturates while increasing their efficacy for the prevention and treatment of *both* heart disease and the fat dependent cancers and, presumably, all the other symptomatic co-diseases comprising the MDS.

THE CLINICAL PICTURE

Hoffer and I have independently observed *(20,21,39)* that today's schizophrenia cannot be distinguished from the dementia of pellagra. Moreover, when today's diseases are viewed clinically *as a group,* the collective picture strongly resembles chronic mixtures of the classical B vitamin deficiency diseases, especially pellagra and beriberi, which often do not show pathognomonic signs such as Casal's collar or all three D's in any one patient.

A review *(20,21)* of the classical literature of about 1900, shows that pellagra routinely produced symptomatic problems which are clinically indistinguishable from today's major illnesses *(20,21)*. Thus, today's schizophrenia, manic depression, and neuroses cannot be distinguished clinically from the pellagrous "dementias" of 1900.

The diarrhea of classical pellagra actually consisted of (1) diarrhea *or* constipation *or* their alternation unaccompanied by other findings except for (2) distention and grumbling and (3) discomfort, i.e., it was "functional." Any two of these three problems now constitute the diagnostic criteria for what is now called "irritable bowel syndrome," "spastic colon" or "mucous colitis," the single most prominent disease seen by gastroenterologists, occupying fully 30% of their practices today.

The chronic form of the "dermatitis" of classical pellagra included dandruff and other drying and scaling xerodermatoses, which are so common today that physicians and dandruff advertisers alike dismiss them as part of the normal human condition, although any veterinarian encountering an animal colony with a similar incidence of problems would know he had a nutritional crisis.

Pellagra also commonly produces tinnitus, fatigue, immune and other idiosyncratic problems, while beriberi produces everything from heart disease to its own variations of the psychoses and neuropathies.

A PILOT CLINICAL TEST
OF THE FATTY SUBSTRATE PELLAGRA-BERIBERI HYPOTHESIS

I have reported elsewhere on the impressive response during a three-year clinical pilot study of forty-four chronic, steady-baseline, previously nonresponding nonplacebo reactors having a large variety of illnesses treated by ω3-EFA supplementation using food grade linseed oil (LSO), which, unlike fish oils, influences all desaturases and, prior to World War II, was a traditional Nordic cooking oil (60% ω3, 20% ω6) *(20,21)*. Conditions permitting, safflower oil (<0.5% ω3, 70% ω6) was used as a control, many cases being repeatedly cycled between these two oils over months.

There has been striking *concomitant* amelioration of a large variety of major mental and physical symptomatic ailments as the *specific* result of adding linseed oil to previously incomplete supplementation regimens including dandruff, arthritis, irritable bowel syndrome, tinnitus, sleeping disturbances, chronic infections, benign prostatic hypertrophy, allergies both food and airborne, discoid lupus, neuralgias, normalization of blood pressure in both directions and others (20,21). Immune system correction has been particularly striking along with reduced cold sensitivity and easier weight control. Severe long-term but remitting (brain competent) schizophrenia and manic-depressive cases have responded impressively. Evidently, therefore, these are all expressions of a highly pleomorphic and idiosyncratic statistical syndrome, even as with classical pellagra and beriberi.

THERAPEUTIC RECOMMENDATIONS

The risk costs of inaction make it imprudent to wait for the niceties of a multimillion dollar ten-year government sponsored study before making the following *no-risk* public recommendations:

(1) Consume more ω3 and less ω6-EFA by reducing beef (keep it lean) and increasing consumption of northern beans (common, red, kidney, navy, pinto) and vegetables cooked *al dente,* chicken, (traditional) pork and one-half to one pound per week of fatty fish (blue, tuna, haddock, rock, mullet, albacore, mussels, mackerel, salmon, trout, oysters). Try kippered herring or smoked salmon (lox) for breakfast (Japanese per capita fish consumption is six times ours). A teaspoon of flaxseed (30% linseed oil) spread over cereal is a dietary tradition in Northern Europe as well as classical Greece and Rome, while wheat germ (as breakfast cereal) is also very high in ω3-EFA. Keep total fats to 35%, ω6, about 6–8% and ω3-EFA about 1–2% of calories and control use of partially hydrogenated food oils and margarines. In the North, at least, use indigenous *nonhydrogenated* soybean, walnut, wheat germ, chestnut, hazelnut, and linseed oils in place of southern cottonseed, sunflower, peanut, safflower, corn, and olive oils or products containing them. Return to butter, used sparingly. Refractory cases may be overwhelmed by covert food antigens, requiring elimination-provocation and chemical diets (Vivonex) properly supplemented per above. When using purified oils in tablespoon daily doses for therapeutic purposes, use supplements to replace stripped-out oil-insoluble B and C vitamins, selenium, and possibly cysteine-methionine, all taken in divided doses with meals or, whenever possible, in time-release form. The regimen is an updated form of the once common use of cod liver oil supplements. For prophylatic purposes take one teaspoon daily of linseed oil, cod liver oil, or somatic fish oil. Because of vitamin A toxicity, avoid cod liver oil megadoses.

(2) Use unprocessed foods high in fiber, e.g., stone-ground cereals labelled more than 2% fiber. Lower cholesterol and sugar intake. Try an artificial sweetener, if necessary. Find the ratio of meat to vegetables that makes one feel best. Take a routine premeal mixed fruit-vegetable-cereal fiber cocktail: 1 part hydrophilic gel fiber (serum cholesterol–lowering) and 4 parts miller's bran (better stool bulking) plus yogurt to suit (seeds the gut with favorable aerobes). Adjust amount (ca. 1 tablespoon) at each routine meal to obtain the normal floating odorless coil BM. Fiber also suppresses appetite and, with wheat germ, reconstitutes today's refined wheat products.

(3) Because of strong coupling of exercise to fat metabolism and atheroma formation *(32),* in the absence of health problems, one should *work up over months* to mild continuous always *enjoyable* aerobic exercise, one-half to one hour every other day, allowing talk over sustained breathlessness and never pushed to fatigue. Vigorous walking, walk-jogging, swimming, cycling, aerobic dancing, etc. are most practical. Intermittent sports do not produce the cardiovascular training effect, which begins only after ten minutes of continuous moderate breathlessness.

(4) Because of strong coupling of stress to steroid-fat metabolism, via Selye's adaptation syndrome, try to optimize this life-style factor to obtain the supersynergistic effect. Details of the supplement regimen for active illness have been given elsewhere *(20,21).*

(5) For illness and a nominal 150 pounds add to the above 1 teaspoon linseed oil at each meal, working up to as much as 1 tablespoon tid or the toleration limit; a one-a-day multivit/multimin (with selenium); 1–2 grams calcium. Continue for four to six months then taper off to zero or maintenance dose or try fish oil concentrate like Maxepa. MegaEFA may produce a beneficial fat, cholesterol, and isomer flush as well as restore normal ω3 EFA levels. Long-

term oil toxicity effects often resemble the original deficiency problems and also include sleepiness, general muscle aching or tendonitis, superficial peeling of finger tips, or roughening of heel skin or knuckles, which may be compensated by increased vitamin E, selenium, or calcium intake. These problems can also be caused, synergistically, by excesses of the other essential nutrients. Corresponding to the symmetrical (bell-shaped) deficiency-toxicity picture, treatment often normalizes BP, serum fats, etc. from both directions. Travel versions are available as LSO capsules, bran-yogurt tablets and bars.

DISCUSSION AND RECOMMENDATIONS

Medically oriented, orthodox nutritionists can be defined as those who say that we are the best fed people in history and that the function of nutrition is to support primary medical treatment. Reform nutritionists are those who say that while we are the best fed people in history we are also the most malnourished and that the function of nutrition is to provide the primary treatment for today's major illnesses, because they are mainly of nutritional origin, the function of medicine being to supply crisis-intervention care in support of nutritional therapy.

Starting in the early 1950s, three lines of reform nutrition research each separately indicated that the modern diet is seriously distorted and may account for many or most of our major illnesses in modernized societies. C. L. Cleave and the British fiber theorists (22) demonstrated that dietary fiber is an essential nutrient, that it is severely deficient in the regular diet, and that it is causally related to various bowel and bowel-related systemic illnesses. A. Hoffer and his colleagues (39) showed that many of our major illnesses, including schizophrenia, can be viewed as vitamin-resistant forms of pellagra and beriberi related to dietary modification together with genetic susceptibility. H. M. Sinclair (40) provided evidence that ω3-EFA deficiencies and excess saturated fat consumption are related to cardiovascular disease, a view now augmented by the Heart and Cancer panels, both of which find dietary fats to be the primary links to illnesses as disparate as heart disease and certain major cancers (1,2).

During this same time, there has been growing recognition by independent epidemiologists that a wide variety of the major illnesses of modernized societies are new or newly prominent and are related to dietary factors (41) rather than to increased diagnostic and therapeutic successes of modern medicine, uncovering heretofore obscure diseases.

The analysis of national food consumption data presented here shows that 70% of our food is now processed or exotic and that this has seriously distorted every essential nutrient family while at the same time significantly increasing the antinutrient load.

When analyzed biochemically, all these findings form a coherent biochemical and clinical picture, because all 50 of our essential conutrients, as well as the antinutrients, are part of a coherent biochemical reaction system—the fundamental reaction of nutrition—which constitutes the front end of our intermediary metabolism which has been delegated evolutionarily to lower sectors of the food chain. It follows that people in modernized societies today, living on a massively distorted dietary base, are at risk for a new kind of subtle but deadly unrecognized synergistic malnutrition—the modern malnutrition—now evidently constituting our primary public health hazard.

Biochemical analysis further indicates that these multiple synergistic dietary modifications can interact synergistically to produce a new diagnostic variant of the classical B vitamin deficiency diseases which once decimated entire populations in both the East and West during the nineteenth century. In particular, I propose that the traditional illnesses be redefined as catalytic B-vitamin type pellagra and beriberi and that we now recognize, in addition, a fat-centered substrate and mixed—deficiency-toxicity—pellagra-beriberi variant of the classical forms, these being the likely cause of what should be recognized as true Modernization Disease *Syndrome* (MDS) now accounting for the bulk of illness.

In fact, the synergy is well established in one small area by the fact that supplements from the three pioneering reform groups cited above—fiber, ω-3 EFA, and niacin—can each alone reduce elevated serum cholesterol. Consequently, concurrent deficiencies, which are now common as the result of the modern dietary distortions, can account for the prevalence of this problem and, conversely, combined supplements of all three essential nutrients will provide the general solution to the problem, provided we also correct the distorted modern diet causing the problem in the first place.

Therefore, contrary to present teaching, Goldberger and Takaki-Eijkmann may have solved only the single food factor, nonsynergistic B-vitamin–sensitive, *catalytic* form of pellagra and beriberi while leaving unrecognized and uncorrected the now dominant vitamin-resistant "Hoffer pellagra-beriberi" variant resulting from a synergistic malnutrition caused by multiple interacting food modifications which presents as a fatty *substrate* or compound (substrate-catalyst-modulator-antinutrient) pellagra-beriberiform illness, the well known idiosyncracy and pleomorphicity of such illnesses misleading the medical profession into thinking it is dealing with dozens of new unrelated illnesses requiring dozens of new specialties.

Because some estimates make the modernization disease group the dominant health problem in modernized societies, these matters should be tested promptly by conducting, under national auspices, an entirely new kind of controlled multifactorial diagnostic and synergistic nutritional therapeutic *interdisease concordance study in man,* which, for the first time, cuts across specialty and even extraclinical boundaries. There should also be conducted primate life cycle tests of the *synergistic* safety and efficacy of the entire food base, placing one-half of a colony of monkeys on the same *total supermarket diet and life-style* on which dietarily modernized man lives. Given the results of Table 2, we may freely predict that the experimental animals will develop all the modern diseases in a few years and recover under nutritional therapy, whenever the damage is not irreversible.

We have been through all this once before, when orthodox nutritionists and the medical profession tolerated massive food refining and other dietary modifications without competent testing, the result of which was the original B-vitamin plagues of 1800–1900. Because we have never outlawed the original refining practices and, indeed, have extended them in many new ways, we are evidently going through a related problem all over again and must conclude that these recurring problems are the result of deep structural problems in the organization of health care, research, and regulation.

The origin of the problem lies in the fact that health care is monopolized by a high tech, high cost, high risk, crisis-intervention oriented allomedical profession, which has an economic as well as a chauvinistic conflict of interest with respect to orthomedical practice using orthotherapy based on orthopharmaceuticals, i.e., our primary pharmacology consisting of natural products including especially essential nutrients. While orthodox allomedicine should have a technical monopoly on dangerous allopharmaceutical agents and other high tech methods, it should not monopolize, as it does, the entire domain of health practice, health regulation, and health research, for this is rather like putting the fox in charge of the chicken coop in view of the fact that the bulk of illnesses today is not medical in nature at all, except by default, but, in the first instance, involves life-style factors—problems of the kitchen and the farm and not the clinic and laboratory.

To correct this unjustified monopoly, we should, as I have suggested elsewhere *(42)* create a new primary health care profession specializing in low cost, low tech, low risk orthomedical treatment and prevention using agents and procedures under control of the patient. The motto of the primary health care profession—the modern hygienist—should be "Primary health care keeps the doctor away." For exactly the same reason, the FDA should be legislatively divided into the FA and DA, with reform and not orthodox nutritionists or physicians heading the Food Administration. Similarly, NIH should be divided into NIH-Medical and NIH-Nutrition, the enabling acts of these new institutions indicating that they have been separated to provide a competitive two-component health care industry, so as to end the current allomedical monopoly, which has failed to provide reasonable health care at reasonable cost for the many modern illnesses which are now putting our people and our nation at risk.

TABLE 2 REFERENCES

(1) Rudin, D. O., Felix, C., with Schrader, C. *The Omega-3 Phenomenon: The Nutritional Breakthrough of the '80s.* New York: Rawson Associates, 1987.

(2) Natvig, H. *et al.* "A Controlled Study of the Effect of Linolenic Acid on the Incidence of Coronary Artery Disease." *Scand. J. Clin. Lab. Invest.* 22:(suppl 5):1–20, 1968.

Dohan, F. C. "Wartime Changes in Hospital Admissions for Schizophrenia. *Acta Psychiat. Scand.* 42:1–23, 1966.

(3) Owren, P. A. "Coronary Thrombosis: Its Mechanism and Possible Prevention by Linolenic Acid." *Ann. Int. Med.* 63:167–84, 1965.

(4) Bagchi, K., Halder, K. and Chowdhury, S. R. "The Etiology of Phrynoderma." *Am. J. Clin. Nutr.* 7:251–8, 1959.

(5) Insull, W. Jr., *et al.* "Studies of Japanese and American Men: Comparisons of Fatty Acid Compositions of Adipose Tissue."*J. Clin. Invest.* 48:1313–27, 1969.

(6) Bang, H. O. *et al.* "The Composition of Food Consumed by Greenland Eskimos." *Acta Med. Scand.* 200:69–73, 1976.

(7) Reed, S. A. "Dietary Source of ω3 Eicosapentaenoic Acid." *Lancet* 2:739–40, 1979.

Annual Report of the National Food Survey Committee, *Household Food Consumption and Expenditure:* 1973, etc. Her Majesty's Stationery Office, London.

(8) Holman, R. T., Johnson, S., and Hatch, T. F. "A Case of Human Linolenic Acid Deficiency Involving Neurological Abnormalities." *Am. J. Clin. Nutr.* 35:617–23, 1982.

(9) Fiennes, R. N., Sinclair, A. J., and Crawford, M. A. "Essential Fatty Acid Studies in Primates: Linolenic Acid Requirements of Capuchins." *J. Med. Primat.* 2:155–69, 1973.

(10) Lamptey, M. S., and Walker, B. L "A Possible Essential Role for Dietary Linolenic Acid in the Development of the Young Rat. *J. Nutr.* 106:86–93, 1976.

TEXT REFERENCES

1. Grobstein, C., NAS/NRC. *Diet, Nutrition and Cancer.* Washington, D. C.: National Academy Press 1982.

2. Grundy, S. M., *et al.* "Rationale of the Diet-Heart Statement of the American Heart Association." Report of the Nutrition Committee, American Heart Association. *Circulation,* 65:839A–54A, April, 1982.

3. Lucas, C. P., and Power, L. "Dietary Fat Aggravates Active Rheumatoid Arthritis." *Clinical Res.* 29:754A, 1981.

4. Goldyne, M. E., and Stobo, J. D. "Immunoregulatory Role of Prostaglandins and Related Lipids." *CRC Critical Reviews in Immunology,* 2:189–223, 1981.

5. Editorial. "Prostaglandins and Immunity." *Lancet* 1:24–5, 1981.

6. Horrobin, D. F. *The Prostaglandins: Physiology, Pharmacology and Clinical Aspects.* St. Albans, VT: Eden, 1978 (p. 242).

7. Weissmann, G. "Release of Mediators of Inflammation." *Prost. & Thera.* 6(2):1–6, 1981.

8. Meade, C. J., and Mertin, J. "Fatty Acids and Immunity." *Adv. Lipid Res.* 16:127–65, 1978.

9. Ebihara, K., *et al.* "Effect of Konjac Mannan on Plasma Glucose and Insulin Responses in Young Men." *Nutr. Rep. Int'l.* 23:577–83, 1981.

10. Honigman, G., *et al.* "Influence of Diet Rich in Linolenic Acid in Diabetics." *Diabetol.* 23:175, 1982.

11. Houtsmuller, A. J., *et al.* "Favorable Influence of Linoleic Acid on the Progression of Diabetic Micro- and Macroangiopathy." *Nutr. Metab.* 1(Supp 24):105–18, 1980.

12. Dodson, P. M., *et al.* "High-Fibre and Low-Fat Diets in Diabetes Mellitus." *Br. J. Nutr.* 46:289–94, 1981.

13. Singer, P., *et al.* "Decrease of Eicosapentaenoic Acid in Fatty Liver of Diabetic Subjects." *Prost. Med.* 5:183–200, 1980.

14. Hansen, A. E., *et al.* "Eczema and Essential Fatty Acid." *Am. J. Dis. Child.* 73:1–18, 1947.

15. Bower, B. O., and Newsholme, E. A. "Treatment of Idiopathic Polyneuritis by a Polyunsaturated Fatty Acid Diet." *Lancet*. 1:583–5, 1978.
16. Lamptey, M. S., and Walker, B. L. "A Possible Essential Role for Dietary Linolenic Acid in the Development of the Young Rat." *J. Nutr.* 106:86–93, 1976.
17. Fiennes, R. N., Sinclair, A. J., and Crawford, M. A. "Essential Fatty Acid Studies in Primates: Linolenic Acid Requirement of Capuchins." *J. Med. Primat.* 2:155–69, 1973.
18. Obi, F. O., and Nwanze, E. A. C. "Fatty Acid Profiles in Mental Disease." *J. Neurol. Sci.* 43:447–54, 1979.
    Dohan, F. C., *et al.* "Schizophrenia: Variations in Prevalence Rates vs Differences in Cereal Grain Consumption." *Soc. Biol. Psychiat.* Meeting. Sept. 1980.
    Dohan, F. C. "Wartime Changes in Hospital Admissions for Schizophrenia." *Acta Psychiatr. Scand.* 42:1–23, 1966.
    Torrey, E. F. *Schizophrenia and Civilization*, Northvale, NJ: Jason Aronson, 1980.
    Page, L. B., Damon, A., and Moellering, R. C. "Antecedents of Cardiovascular Disease in Six Solomon Islands Societies." *Circulation* 49:1132–46, 1974.
19. Chase, H. P., *et al.* "Intravenous Linoleic Acid Supplementation in Children with Cystic Fibrosis. *Pediat.* 64:207–13, 1979.
    Harper, T. B., *et al.* "Essential Fatty Acid Deficiency in Rabbit as a Model of Nutritional Impairment in Cystic Fibrosis." *Am. Rev. Respir. Dis.* 126:540–7, 1982.
20. Rudin, D. O. "The Dominant Diseases of Modernized Societies as Omega-3 Essential Fatty Acid Deficiency Syndrome: Substrate Beriberi." *Med. Hypotheses* 8:17–47, 1982.
    Rudin, D. O. "The Major Psychoses and Neuroses as Omega-3 Essential Fatty Acid Deficiency Syndrome: Substrate Pellagra." *Biol. Psychiat.* 16(9):837–50, 1981.
    Rudin, D. O. "The Three Pellagras." *J. Orthomol. Psychiatry* 12(2):91–110, 1983.
21. Rudin, D. O. *The Omega-3 Phenomenon: The Nutritional Breakthrough of the '80s.* New York: Rawson Associates, 1987.
22. Cleave, T. L. *The Saccharine Disease: The Master Disease of Our Time*. New Canaan, CT: Keats, 1975.
    Heaton, K. W. *Bile Salts in Health and Disease*. New York: Churchill Livingstone, 1972.
    Reddy, B. S. "Dietary Fiber and Colon Cancer." *Can. Med. Assoc. J. 123*:850–6, 1980.
23. Hill, E. G., *et al.* "Perturbation of the Metabolism of EFA by Dietary Partially Hydrogenated Vegetable Oil." *PNAS* 79:953–7, 1982.
    Rosenthal, M. D., and Doloresco, M. A. "Effects of Transfatty Acids on Fatty Acyl Delta-5 Desaturation by Human Skin Fibroblasts." *Lipids* 19:869–74, 1984.
    Deschrijver, R., and Privett, O. S. "Energetic Efficiency and Mitochondrial Function in Rats Fed Trans-fatty Acids. *J. Nutrition* 114:1183–91, 1984.
24. King, J. C., *et al.* "Evaluation and Modification of the Basic Four Food Guide." *J. Nutr. Ed.* 10:27–9, 1978.
    Guthrie, H. A., and Scheer, J. C. "Nutritional Adequacy of Self-selected Diets That Satisfy the Four Food Groups Guide." *J. Nutr. Ed.* 13:46–9, 1981.
25. Ayala, S., Brenner, R. R., and Dumm, C. G. "Effect of Polyunsaturated Fatty Acids of the Alpha-Linolenic Series on Rat Testicle Development." *Lipids* 12:1017–24, 1977.
    Dumm, I. N. T., *et al.* "Effect of Catecholamines and Beta Blockers on Linoleic Acid Desaturation Activity." *Lipids* 13:649–52, 1978.
    Dumm, I. N. T., *et al.* "Comparative Effect of Glucagon, cAMP and Epinephrine on Desaturation and Elongation of Linoleic Acid by Rat Liver Microsomes." *Lipids* 11:833–6, 1976.
    Dumm, I. N. T. "Effect of Glucocorticoids on the Oxidative Desaturation of Fatty Acids by Rat Liver Microsomes." *J. Lipid Res.* 20:834–9, 1979.
26. Kramsch, D. M., *et al.* "Reduction of Coronary Artery Atherosclerosis by Moderate Exercise in Monkeys on an Atherogenic Diet." *NEJM* 305:1483–9, 1981.
27. Selye, H. *Stress in Health and Disease*. Stoneham, MA: Butterworth, 1976.
28. Saynor, R. "Effects of Omega-3 Fatty Acids on Serum Lipids." *Lancet* 2:696–7, 1984.
    Bronte-Stewart, B., *et al.* "Effects of Feeding Different Fats on Serum Cholesterol Level." *Lancet* 1:521–7, 1956.

Owren, P. A. "Coronary Thrombosis: Its Mechanism and Possible Prevention by Linolenic Acid." *Ann. Int. Med.* 63:167–84, 1965.

Sinclair, H. M. "Valedictory Address." *Prog. Fd. Nutr. Sci.* 4:131–4, 1980.

Phillipson, B. E., *et al.* "Reduction of Plasma Lipids, Lipoproteins and Apoproteins by Dietary Fish Oils in Patients with Hypertriglyceridemia." *NEJM* 312:1210–16, 1985.

Kromhout, D., *et al.* "The Inverse Relation Between Fish Consumption and 20 Year Mortality from Coronary Heart Diseases." *NEJM* 312:1205–9, 1985.

29. Kritchevsky, D. "Fiber, Lipids and Arteriosclerosis." *Am. J. Clin. Nutr.* 31:S65–S74, 1978.

Terasawa, F., *et al.* "Effects of Konjac Flour on Blood Lipids in Elderly Subjects." *Eiyogaku Zasshi* 37:23–8, 1979.

Kiriyama, S., *et al.* "Hypocholesterolemic Activity and Molecular Weight of Konjac Mannan." *Nutrition Reports International.* 6:231–6, 1972.

30. Hunninghake, D. B. "Pharmacologic Therapy for the Hyperlipidemic Patient." *Am. J. Med.* 74(5A):19–22, 1983.

Hotz, W. "Nicotinic Acid and Its Derivatives: A Short Survey." *Adv. in Lipid Res.* 20:195–217, 1983.

31. Birch, T. W. "The Relation Between Vitamin B_6 and the unsaturated Fatty Acid Factor." *JBC* 124:775–93, 1938.

Quackenbush, F. W., *et al.* "Linoleic Acid, Pyridoxine and Pantothenic Acid in Rat Dermatitis." *J. Nutr.* 24:225–34, 1942.

Evans, H. M., and Lepkovsky, S. "The Sparing Action of Fat on Vitamin B. *JBC* 96:165–77, 1932.

Bhat, K. S., and Belavady, B. "Biochemical Studies in Phrynoderma." *Am. J. Clin. Nutr.* 20:386–92, 1967.

Ellis, J., *et al.* "Clinical Results of a Crossover Treatment with Pyridoxine and Placebo of the Carpal Tunnel Syndrome." *Am. J. Clin. Nutr.* 32:2040–6, 1979.

Folkers, K., *et al.* "Biochemical Evidence for a Deficiency of Vitamin B_6 in Carpal Tunnel Syndrome." *PNAS* 75:3410–12, 1978.

Folkers, K., *et al.* "Enzymology of the Response of the Carpal Tunnel Syndrome to Riboflavin and to Combine Riboflavin and Pyridoxine." *PNAS* 81:7076–78, 1984.

32. Schramm, T. "Effect of Fatty Acids on Carcinogenesis." *Wiss. Z. Humboldt.* 11:184–5, 1962.

Karmali, R. A., *et al.* "Effect of Omega-3 Fatty Acids on Growth of a Rat Mammary Tumor." *JNCI* (US) 73:457–61, 1984.

33. Abraham, S., and Hillyard, L. A. "Effect of Dietary 18-Carbon Fatty Acids on Growth of Transplantable Mammary Adenocarcinoma in Mice." *JNCI* (US) 71:601–5, 1983.

Chan, P. C., *et al.* "Effects of Different Dietary Fats on Mammary Carcinogenesis." *Cancer Res.* 43:1079–83, 1983.

34. Horvath, P. M., and Ip, C. "Synergistic Effect of Vitamin E and Selenium in the Chemoprevention of Mammary Carcinogenesis in Rats." *Cancer Res.* 43:5335–41, 1983.

Witting, C. H., *et al.* "The Tumor-Protective Effect of Selenium in an Experimental Model." *J. Cancer Res. Clin. Oncol.* 104:109–13, 1982.

Young, E. O., and Milner, J. A. "Influence of Zinc and Selenium Intake on DMBA Induced Mammary Tumors in Rats." *J. Nutr.* 112:R30, 1982.

35. Ip, C., and Sinha, D. K. "Enhancement of Mammary Tumors by Selenium Deficiency in Rats with High Polyunsaturated Fat Intake." *Cancer Res.* 41:31–4, 1981.

36. Goldyne, M. E., and Stobo, J. D. "Immunoregulatory Role of Prostaglandins and Related Lipids." *CRC Critical Reviews in Immunology* 2:189–223, 1981.

Hansen, H. S. "EFA Supplemented Diet Increases Renal Excretion of PGE2 and Water in EFA Deficient Rats." *Lipids* 16:849–54, 1981.

Prickett, J. D., *et al.* "Dietary Enrichment with Polyunsaturated Fatty Acid Eicosapentaenoic Acid Prevents Proteinuria and Prolongs Survival in NZB x NZW F1 Mice. *J. Clin. Inves.* 68:556–9, 1981.

37. Spallholz, J. E. "Anti-inflammatory, Immunologic and Carcinostatic Attributes of Selenium in Experimental Animals." *Adv. Exp. Med. and Biol.* 135:43–62, 1981.
38. Trudel J. L. "The Fat/Fiber Antagonism in Experimental Colon Carcinogenesis." *Surgery* (US), 94:691–6, 1983.
39. Hoffer, A., and Walker, M. *Orthomolecular Nutrition.* New Canaan, CT: Keats, 1978.
40. Sinclair, H. M. "Valedictory Address." *Prog. Fd. Nutr. Sci.* 4:131–4, 1980.
41. Hegstedt, D. M. Testimony. Hearing, Senate Select Committee on the Relation of Nutrition to Disease. *Congressional Record,* 1976.
42. Rudin, D. O. "Call for a National Conference to Form the American Federation of Primary Health Care Societies." *J. Orthomol. Psychiatry* 13(1):25–26, 1984.

Index

Italic type denotes recipes

A

AA (arachidonic acid), 11
Acne, 53, 54–55, 114, 241
Acrodermatitis enteropathica, 56
Acrodynia, 105
Adolescence, 35–36
Aerobic exercise, 160, 163–68, 241
Aging, 114, 234–37
Aging disease, 241
Agoraphobia, 77–78
AIDS, 88
Alcohol consumption, 60
Alcoholism, 49, 114
Allergies, 3, 78
  common, 225–26
  elimination diets for, 227, 228
  substitutions due to, 107
  testing for, 227
Allergy addiction, 161
Almond oil, 24
Alopecia, 241
Alopecia areata, 53
Alpha linolenic acid (ALA), xiv, 10, 12,
    13, 56, 84, 241
Amenorrhea, 241
Amino acids, 241
Anemia, 61, 114, 241
Angina, 241
Anosmia, 241
Antinutrient, x, 241
  and toxicity, 31–32
Antioxidant, 241
Antisocial behavior, 114
Anxiety-depression, 3
Aorta, 241
Appetite, control of, 161

Apricot kernel oil, 24
Arachidonic acid, 66, 241
Arteriosclerosis, 241
Artery, 241
Arthritis, 3, 45, 61, 101, 114, 226
Aspirin, 113
Asthma, 55
Atherosclerosis, 29, 82, 241
Autism, 72–73, 241
Avocado oil, 24

B

Bacteria, 126, 241
Basic Low-Calorie Brown Sauce, 203
Basic Low-Calorie White Sauce, 203
Beans
  reducing gas potential in, 123
  recipes with, 152, 153
Beef
  Omega EFA in, 124
  recipes with, 194, 196
Benigh prostatic hypertrophy (BPH),
    244–45
Benign, 241
Beriberi, xii, ix, 6, 24, 241
Beta carotene, xi, 241, 244
  deficiency of, 31
Bile acids, 26
Biotin, 100, 101
Black Bean Soup, 223
Blood clotting
  role cf thromboxane in, 85
  slowing of accelerated, 84
Bottle feeding, 69–70
Bowel/bowel-related diseases, xii
Bowel training, of toddler, 71

Brain
  and dietary deficiencies, 81
  role of essential fatty acids in, 20
  role of Omega-3 in development of,
      66–67
Breast cancer, 61
Breast-feeding, 68–69, 230
  counter-indications for, 69
  and increased food intake, 229
Broccoli, Scrambled Eggs with, 219
Broiled Falafel Patties, 152
Broiled Fish, 150
Brown adipose tissue, 241
Brown fat, 159–60, 241
Bruising, 114
Burkitt, D. P., 26
Burkitt, Denis, 4
Bursitis, 44–45, 61, 114, 242
Butter, Diet, 205

C

Caffeine, 242
Calcium, 91, 103
  deficiency of, 104, 105
Calorie, 242
  and weight maintenance, 171
Cancer, x, 3, 29, 114, 242
  role of diet with, 38
Cancer cells, 233–34
Capillary, 242
Carbohydrate, 242
  RDA of, 140–41
Carcinogen, 26, 242
Cardiopulmonary training effect, 164
Cardiovascular disease, 114, 242
  and Omega-3 EFA deficiency, xii
  and Omega-3 EFA therapy, 47
  role of diet with, 37
Carotene, 94, 242
Carpal tunnel syndrome, 242
Cataracts, 114
Celiac disease, 3, 226
Cellulose, 26, 242
Cereal and grains, in an Omega diet, 119,
      121
Cheese Soufflé, 152
Chelate, 242
Chestnut oil, 95
Chicken Salad, 201
Cholesterol, 242
  and EFA, 16, 56–57
  lowering of, 26

Cleave, T. L., xi–xii, 4, 26
Cobalt, deficiency of, 31
Coconut oil, 9, 22, 24
Cod liver oil supplements, xiv
Cofactors, 20, 99
  deficiencies in, 39
Cold climates, fats from, 12
Cold-climate
  ultrapolyunsaturates, xiv
Coleslaw, Creamy, 201
Colic, in infants, 70
Colitis, 107
Collagen, 242
Constipation, 87
Conutrients, 242
Copper, 103–4
  deficiency of, 31
  toxic effects from, 104
Corn oil, 9, 22, 24, 84, 95
Cortisone, 113
Cottage Cheese Grill Maxine, 194
Cottage Cheese Soufflé, 217
Cottonseed oil, 9, 22, 95
Creamed Tuna on Toast, 150
Creamy Coleslaw, 201
Curried Eggs, 152–53
Cuticle, 242
Cyanocobalamin. *See* Vitamin B$_{12}$
Cysteine, 104
  dietary deficiency of, 31
Cystic fibrosis, 3, 114
Cystitis, 47
Cysts, flare-up of, 111

D

Dairy products, choice of, 132
Dandruff, 114
Davis, Adelle, 4
Dehydroepiandrosterone (DHEA), 160
Depression, 115, 242
Dermatitis, 54–55, 242
Dermis, 242
Desocyribonucleic acid (DNA), 242
Desserts
  choice of, 133
  recipes with, 206–7
DHA (docosahexaenoic acid), 11, 12, 40,
      64, 66, 68–69, 84
Diabetes, xii, 3, 115, 242
  and diet, 38–40
Diet
  avoiding sugar in, 128, 129

effect of, on health, x, 3–4
length of, 171
need to stick with, 93
plateaus in, 160, 169
proportions of foods in, 8
tips for, 173–74
Dietary EFA, disruption of, 20–21
Dietary fiber. *See* Fiber
Dietary malnutrition, 235
Diet Butter, 205
Digestive system
effect of fiber on, 29, 106
effect of prostaglandins on, 17
role of Omega-3 in improving disor-
ders of, 18
Diphtheria, 3
Discoid lupus, 54–55
Disease
correlation of diet with, 3–4
development of, 33–42
Diuretic, 242
Diverticulitis, xii, 242
Docosahexaenoic acid (DHA), 242
Double bond, 242
Drinks, choice of, 133
Dry beriberi, 6
Dupuytren's contracture, 115
Dyspareunia, 115, 242

E

Early childhood, Omega deficiency in,
70–74
Eczema, 52, 54–55, 242
Edema, 242
EFA (essential fatty acids), x, 243
and brain function, 20
and cholesterol, 16
composition of food oils, 23–24
conversion of, by B vitamins, xi
deficiencies in, 30
dietary need for, 10–11
functions of, 11
normalizing intake, 127
role of, in body, 15–16
sources of, 247–55
toxic effects from, 104
Efamol, 95n, 110
EFA-prostaglandin connection, 17
and heart disease, 37
Eggs, recipes with, 152–53, 219
Eijkmann, xiv
Elevated serum fats, xii

Emotional stability, 44
Endocrine problems, 115
Endometriosis, 111
Enzymes, 19, 99, 236, 242
EPA (eicosapentaenoic acid), 11, 12,
68–69, 84, 121
Esophagus, 243
Essential fatty acids (EFA). *See* EFA
Essential fatty acid-prostaglandin
system, xi
Estrogen, 243
Estrogen replacement therapy, 64
Evening primrose oil, xv, 72, 110–11
Exercise, 13, 20
aerobic, 160, 163–68, 241
importance of, 31, 93
strengthening, 167–68
stretching, 165–67
Eye problems, and diabetes, 40

F

Facials, 60
Fast foods, xiii
Fats
body uses for, 9
composition of, 9
dietary reputation of, 8
in human nutrition, 9–11
polyunsaturated, 10
recommended consumption of, 8
RDA of, 140–41
saturated, 9, 10
as source of energy, 9
unsaturated, 9, 10
Fat-soluble vitamins, 9
Fatty acids, 10
RDA of, 140
Fettuccine al Marco, 154
Fiber, 26, 99, 243
in baby's diet, 232
buying in bulk, 106
and cancer, 38
deficiencies in, xii, 28–29, 31
and diabetes, 39–40
intake level of, 27–28
need for in diet, x, 26–27
and need for Omega-3, 29
RDA of, 140
Fiber Cocktail, 29, 91, 129
Fiber cofactors, 20, 105–7
Fiber supplements, xii, 93
Filet Mignon and Mushrooms, 194

Fish
  choice of, 132
  recipes with, 150
  as source of Omega-3, 125
Fish oils, 12–14
  balancing with, 110
  benefits from, 84–85
  as source of Omega-3, 4
  supplements, xv
"Flaky paint" dermatitis, 243
Flaxseed, 13
Fluoride, 129
Floacin, 100, 101
Follicular keratosis, 54
Food and Nutrition Board of the Na-
      tional Academy of Science, 8
Food-grade linseed oil, xiv
  as source of Omega-3, 4
Food groups, in the Omega diet, 119–29
Food oils, 23
Food processing, as nutritional problem,
      xii-xiii, x, 4
Formication, 243
Fowl. *See* Poultry
Free-choice Omega diets, 175
Free radical, 243
French Apple Yogurt, 224
French Dressing, 200
French Toast, 217
Fruit group, in the Omega diet, 119,
      120–21
"Funny fats," 21, 30

G

Galli, C., 67
Gallstones, xii
Ganglia, 17
Garbanzo and Cheese Loaf, 218
Gastritis, 243
Gastrointestinal, 243
Genetics, 30
  and health, 30
  and obesity, 159
GLA (gamma linolenic acid), 11
Glucagon, 38
Glucammannan, 121
Glucose, 243
Gluten allergy, 226
Gourmet-thin Omega Diet
  menus for, 186–92
  recipes for, 193–207
  suggested dishes, 184

weight-loss rules, 185
Great American Experimental Diet,
      238–39
Greek-Style Skillet, 154
Guacamole-Stuffed Tomato, 221

H

Hair problems, 116
Harris, William S., 84
Hay fever, 55
Headache, 61, 115
  and Omega-3 EFA therapy, 46
Healing, 17–18
Health
  effect of diet on, 3–4
  factors which effect, 30–32
Heart disease, 3, 101
  and dietary fats, x
  dietary treatment of, 86
  EFA-prostaglandin link with, 37
  and Omega therapy, 82–86
Heart rate measurement, 164
Hemicellulose, 26
Hemoglobin, 243
Hemorrhoids, 87
Heredity. *See* Genetics
Herpes, 88, 115
High-density lipoprotein (HDL), 243
High serum cholesterol, 116
Hoffer, A., xii, 4, 35, 130
Hoffer pellagra, xii
Hormone, 243
Horrobin, David, 110
Hydrogenated fat, 243
Hydrogenation, xiii, 9, 21, 22
Hydrophilic fibers, 26
Hyperactivity, 3, 72
Hyperglycemia, 243
Hyperlipidemia, 84
Hypertension, 29, 115, 243
  and Omega-3 therapy, 47
Hyperthyroidism, 87
Hypoglycemia, 39, 243
Hypotension, 115, 243

I

Ibuprofen, 113
Ice cream, 207
Immune disorders, 115
  amelioration of, 45–46
  and diet, 41

Immune system, 72–73, 243
  and cancer, 38
  failure of, 45–46
  prenatal development and, 66
Indian Curry, 194
Infant
  feeding of, 68–70
  formula, 69, 230
  starting on solid foods, 231
Infectious diseases, 3
Infertility, 63, 115
Insomnia, 243
Insulin, 38
Insulin effect, 161
Irish Stew, 156
Iron
  deficiency of, 104, 105
  toxic effects from, 104
Irritable bowel syndrome (IBS), xii, 3,
  70, 78, 81, 87, 243
  and Omega-3 EFA therapy, 47–48
Irritable brain sydrome, 81
Irritable esophageal syndrome, 81
Irritable syndrome, 243
Isomers, xiii, 21

J

Jogging program, 165
Joint diseases, 78
Jojoba oil, 58, 59

K

Keratin, 51
Kidney Bean Salad, 222
Kunin, Richard, 109

L

Labels, reading, 131
Lactobacillus acidophilus, 126
Lactones, 32
Lactose, 126, 243
Lactose intolerance, 243
Lamb
  recipes with, 194–95
  Omega EFA in, 125
Lappe, Frances Moore, 124
Laxatives, 93
Lecithin, 99
Legumes
  choice of, 132
  as source of Omega-3, 122–24
Light hydrogenation, 22

Lignin, 26
Linoleic acid, 10, 11, 243
  food sources for, 11
Linolenic acid, 243
Linseed oil, xv, 9, 12–14, 58, 95, 97
  directions for taking, 97, 99
  EFA composition of, 23
  finding correct dosage, 96
  and Omega-3, 12–14
  and problem of rancidity, 95
  selection of, 94–95
  as source of Omega-3, 23
  as supplement, 63
  therapy, 112–13
  topical application of, 47, 113
  and toxicity, 96–97
Lipid-centered malnutrition, x
Lipid deficiency/toxicity syndrome, x
Lipid metabolism, 31
Lipids, 243
Lithium, 79, 80
Lomma Linda's Soylao, 69
Longevity, 233–37
Low-Calorie Cheese Sauce, 204
Low-Calorie Curry Sauce, 204
Low-Carloie French Wine and Cheese
  Sauce, 205
Low-Calorie Maple-Flavored Syrup, 205
Low-density lipoprotein (LDL), 243
Lubriderm, 59

M

Macaroni and Cheese, Baked, 193
Magnesium
  dietary deficiency of, 31
  toxic effects from, 104
Male virility, 64–65
Malignant, 243
Malnutrition
  and hyperactivity, 72
  in infants, 71
  modern, 238
Malnutritional synergy, 267
Manganese, 103–4
Manic-depression, 78–80
Maple-Honey Syrup, 206
Mastiti, 115
Maxepa, 54, 94, 95n, 110
Meat
  choice of, 132
  from the Omega viewpoint, 120
  as source of Omega-3, 124–25

Megadosing, xi
  with B vitamins, 101
Mega-nutrients
  avoiding excessive, 92
  toxicity effects of, 112
Ménière's disease, 81, 87, 243–44
Menopause, 115
  and Omega-3 EFA therapy, 47
  and vaginal secretions after, 64
Menstrual cramps, 63
Mental disorders, types of, 36
Mental health, and Omega-3 therapy,
    76–81, 88
Metabolic malnutrition, 235
Metabolism, 244
  slow down in, and diet plateaus, 160
Methionine, 104
  dietary deficiency of, 31
Middle Eastern Tacos, 218
Migrane headache, 244
  See also Headache
Milk allergy, 226
Milk and diary products, as source of
    Omega-3, 126
Mineral cofactors, 20, 102–5, 108–9, 111
Minerals, RDA of, 139
Mock Sour Cream, 206
Modernization disease syndrome, x, ix,
    72
  as substrate pellagra-beriberi, 263–67
Monosodium glutamate, 226
Monosunsaturated fats, 244
Mousse, Low-Cal Cottage Cheese, 206
Mucous colitis, xii
Multiple sclerosis, 115
Mustard Salad Dressing, 200

N

Nail problems, 115
Natural Ovens, 13
Neo-Mull-Soy liquid, 69
Neuralgia, 87
Neuropathy, 115
Neurosis, 115, 244
Neutroderm, 59
Niacin. *See* Vitamin B$_3$
Nightshades, 226
Nitrates, 226
Nitrite, 226, 244
No-Choice Omega Diet, 175–76
Nonessential fatty acids, 15

Nonhydrogenated high Omega-3 prod-
    ucts, 25
Northern oils, 24–25
Norwegian notch, 33–34, 83
Nutrient depletion, 32
Nutrient interaction, 104–5
Nutrient supplements, 104
Nutrition newspapers/newsletters,
    261–62
Nutritional synergism, xi
Nuts, as source of Omega-3, 122

O

Obesity, 3, 40–41, 116, 244
Olive oil, 24, 95
Omega, 244
Omega-3 EFA, xiv, 9–11, 244
  adjusting dosage, 108
  and cholesterol, 14–15
  and cold climates, 128
  deficiency in, xii, 16
  dietary need for, xi, 4
  difference between Omega-6 EFA and,
    11
  as essential nutrient, 4, 29
  food sources for, 11, 12
  and linseed oil, 12–14, 23
  maintenance of program, 108–9
  potency of, 24
  problem of rancidity, 24
  problem of too much, 111
  and prostaglandins, 18
  research on deficiencies in, 4–5, 34–35
Omega-3 oils, 91
  and climate changes, 109–10
  intake of, 94–99, 127
Omega-3 program, 13
  development of, 23–25
  health benefits from, 43–49
Omega-6 EFA, 9–11, 244
  deficiency of, 16
  difference between Omega-3 EFA and,
    11
Omega-6 oil, ratio of, with Omega-3, 109
Omega diet, 127–29
  advantages of, 137
  antiaging, 233–37
  antiallergy, 225–28
  for babies and toddlers, 231–32
  for mothers and infants, 229–32
  overview of standard, 138–39

recipes for standard, 149–50
RDA of, 139–40
single-dish meals, 150–56
special tips, 151
weekly menus, 141–48
Omega hypoallergenic diet, 94
Omega Mayonnaise, 149, 200
Omega nutrients, 22–25
Omega Oil and Vinegar Salad Dressing,
149
Omega Omelet, 195
Omega Supplemental Program, 238
health benefits from, 44–49
and other nutrients, 100
for overt illness, 91–116
Omega weight loss program
choice of diets, 174–75
free-choice diet, 184
Gourmet-thin Omega Diet, 184–207
menus in, 177–83
and obesity, 158–61
omegafying of diet, 176
phases of, 157–58, 161–76
snacks in, 176
Veggie-thin diet, 175, 208–23
Omelet, Omega, 195
Organ meats, 124
Orthopharmacology, xi
Orthotherapy, 239
Osteoarthritis, 44–45
Osteoporosis, 61, 116, 244
Ovary, 244
Over-the-counter drugs, 113

P

Painter, N.S., 26
Palm kernel oil, 9, 22, 24
Pantothenic acid. *See* Vitamin (B₅)
Pantry, stocking of, 134–36
Paresthesia, 48
Pasteur, Louis, xvi
Peanut oil, 22, 24, 95
Pectin, 244
Pellagra, ix, xii, 17, 56, 244
Peppercorn Steak, 196
Peptic ulcer, xii
Pernicious anemia, 24
Phrynoderma, 54
Phytic acid, 105
Pita, Stuffed, 221
Placebo, 244

Plankton, 121
Platelet, 244
Pneumonia, 3
Polyunsaturated fats, 10, 21–22
Polyunsaturated fatty acid (PUFA), 67,
244
Pork, Omega EFA in, 124–25
Potato Latkes, 153
Poultry
choice of, 132
as source of Omega-3, 125
Premarin, 47, 87
Premature infant, immune system of, 68
Premenstrual syndrome (PMS), 61–64,
87, 101, 116, 244
Prenatal care, 65–67
and increased food intake, 229
and native foods, 74–75
and special diets, 230
Price, Weston A., 73
Primrose oil, 94
Promega, 110
Prostacyclin, 85
Prostaglandins (PG), 11, 16–22, 30, 244
and brain function, 20
and digestive system, 17, 18
and diabetes, 39
EFA connection, 17, 20–21
and healing, 17–18
and Omega-3, 18
and polyunsaturated fats, 21–22
production, 113
role of, 18–20
and trans-fatty acids, 21
and vegetable oils, 22
Prostate, 244–45
Prostate disease, 47
Prostatic hypertrophy, 65, 116
Protein, RDA of, 140–41
Psoriasis, 87, 116
Pyorrhea, 87
Pyridoxine (B₆), 100, 101

Q

Quick-Poached Salmon, 196

R

Ratatouille, 219
Raynaud's disease, 85, 87, 116
Recommended Daily Allowances,
139–41, 245

Red Wine Dressing, 200–201
Reed, J., xii
Reform nutritionists, 4, 239
Relaxation, 93
Renal colic, 87
Retinoic acid, 54–55
Rheumatoid arthritis, 45
Riboflavin. *See* Vitamin B₂
Rice, recipes with, 149, 153, 155
Roman bread, 13
Roman Rice and Beans, 153
Roquefort Dressing, 201

S

Safflower oil, 22, 24, 84, 95
Salad Dressings, 149, 200–1
Salads
    recipes for, 201–2, 221–222
Salmon, recipes for, 193, 196
Salmon oil, 23, 84
Saturated fats, 9, 10, 245
    and disease, 21
Sauces
    recipes for, 203–5, 207
Savory Rice, 155
Scallops, recipes for, 193
Schizophrenia, 3, 245
    role of diet in, 35–36, 76–77
Scrambled Eggs with Broccoli, 219
Scurvy, 245
Seaweed, 121
Seborrheic dermatitis, 108, 245
Seeds, as source of Omega-3, 122
Selenium, xi, xii, 29, 58, 91, 94, 103
    deficiency of, 31
    toxic effects from, 104
Senekote, 93
Sesame oil, 24, 95
Sexually transmitted diseases, 88
Shopping guide, 130–36
Shrimp, recipes for, 149, 197
Sinclair, H. M., xii, 4
Skin
    cells of, 51
    functions of, 50
    monitoring progress through, 107–9
    and Omega-3, 44, 52–57
    problems in, 116
    rules of care, 60
    structure of, 51
    topical program for, 58–60

Slant board technique, 58–59
Smallpox, 3
Smell disorders, 116
Smith, Lendon, 70
Smoking, and skin care, 60
Snacks, 176
Socini, A., 67
Soup, recipes for, 199, 222–23
Sour Cream, Mock, 206
Southern oils, 24–25
Soybean oil, 22, 24, 95
    adding to infant formula, 69
Soylac, 230
Soy oil, 9, 58
Spastic colon, xii
Spinach, recipes for, 202, 220
Spread, recipes for, 224
Steroids, 113
Stew Irish, 156
Stir-Fried Turkey Tenderloins, 196–97
Strengthening exercises, 167–68
Stress, 13, 20
    and health, 31, 41–42
    and need for relaxation, 93
    and obesity, 41, 159
Stretching exercises, 165–67
Stroke, 3, 245
Stuffed Pita, 221
Substrate, 245
Sudden infant death syndrome (SIDS),
    71
Sugar, in diet, 128, 129
Sugar addiction, 161
Sulfites, 226
Sunflower oil, 22, 24
Sunscreens, 60
Svennerholm, Lars, 66
Swiss Cheese Spread, 224
Synergistic malnutrition, ix, 13, 40
Syntex, 69
Syrup, recipes for, 205, 206

T

Tabouli, 220
Tacos, recipes for, 198, 218
Takaki, xiv
Taste disorders, 116
Teeth, effect of diet on, 73–74
Tendonitis, 44–45
Thiamine. *See* Vitamin B₁

Thromboxane, 85
Tinnitus, 78, 81, 116, 245
Toddlers, diet of, 71, 231–32
Tomato, Guacamole-Stuffed, 221
Tostadas, 155
Toxicity
  and antinutrients, 31–32
  from linseed oil, 96–97
Trace minerals, 103–4
  deficiencies in, 31
  RDA of, 139
Trans-fatty acids, 21, 245
Trauma healing, 116
Traveling, and dieting, 93–94
Trowell, H., 26
Tuberculosis, 3
Tuna, recipes for, 150, 198, 202
Turkey, recipes for, 196–97, 199
Type A personality, 30, 245
Typhoid fever, 3
Tyramine, 245

U

Ultrapolyunsaturates, x, 12
Unsaturated fats, 9, 10, 245
Urinary problems, 47

V

Vaginal, 245
Vaginal problems, 63, 64
Varicose veins, 245
Veal Cutlet Romano, 199
Vegetable oils, 22
Vegetables
  choice of, 132
  in the Omega diet, 119, 120–21
  from the sea, 121
Vegetable Salad, 221
Veggie-thin Omega Diet, 208–209
  menus for, 210–16
  pros and cons, 175
  recipes for, 217–24
Vein, 245
Virus, 245
Vision problems, 116
Vitamin(s), 245
  as cofactor, 20, 100–2, 108–9, 111
  deficiencies in, 30–31
  RDA of, 139–40
Vitamin A, xi, 101–2

and acne, 54–55
  toxic effects from, 104
Vitamin antioxidants, xii
Vitamin B, 100–1
  body's need for, 81
  consumption of, x
  deficiencies, ix, 55–56
  EFA connection, 56
Vitamin B$_1$, 100, 101
  deficiency of, 6, 30
Vitamin B$_2$, 100, 101
  deficiency of, 30
Vitamin B$_3$, xii, 100, 101
  and cholesterol, 27
  deficiency of, 7, 30, 56
  toxic effects from 104
Vitamin B$_5$, 100, 101
Vitamin B$_6$, deficiency of, 30
Vitamin B$_{12}$, 100, 101
  deficiency of, 24
Vitamin C, xi, 29, 102
  deficiency of, 31
Vitamin D, toxic effects from, 104
Vitamin E, xi, 29, 58, 59, 102
  deficiency of, 31
  toxic effects from, 104
Vitamin pro-A. *See* Beta-carotene
Vivonex, 227

W

Waldorf Salads, 222
Walking program, 165
Walnut oil, 9, 23, 58, 95
Water
  need for, 129
  RDA of, 139
Watercress Soup, 222–223
Weight, ideal, 169, 170
Weight loss
  charting, 172
  time needed for, 171
Weight-loss diets, fats in, 8
Wet beriberi, 6
Wheat allergy, 226
Wheat germ oil, 9, 23, 58, 95
Wheat-Soy Varnishkes, 156
Women, nutritional needs of, 61–64

X

Xeroderma, 245

Y

Yogurt, French Apple, 224
Yogurt-fiber cocktail, 106
Yo-yo syndrome, 158

Z

Zesty Quick Onion Soup, 199
Zinc, 65, 103–4
    deficiency of, 31, 104, 105
    and EFA connection, 56